9 MONTHS THAT COUNT FOREVER

How your pregnancy diet shapes your baby's future

Also by Jessie Inchauspé

Glucose Revolution
The Glucose Goddess Method

9 MONTHS THAT COUNT FOREVER

How your pregnancy diet shapes your baby's future

JESSIE INCHAUSPÉ
The Glucose Goddess

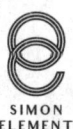

SIMON ELEMENT

New York   Amsterdam/Antwerp   London
Toronto   Sydney/Melbourne   New Delhi

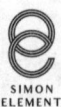
SIMON ELEMENT

An Imprint of Simon & Schuster, LLC
1230 Avenue of the Americas
New York, NY 10020

For more than 100 years, Simon & Schuster has championed authors and the stories they create. By respecting the copyright of an author's intellectual property, you enable Simon & Schuster and the author to continue publishing exceptional books for years to come. We thank you for supporting the author's copyright by purchasing an authorized edition of this book.

No amount of this book may be reproduced or stored in any format, nor may it be uploaded to any website, database, language-learning model, or other repository, retrieval, or artificial intelligence system without express permission. All rights reserved. Inquiries may be directed to Simon & Schuster, 1230 Avenue of the Americas, New York, NY 10020 or permissions@simonandschuster.com.

Copyright © 2026 by Glucose Goddess SAS

The material in this book is for informational purposes only. The action plans presented are based on my understanding of the science, and should not be taken as clinical advice. As each individual situation is unique, you should use proper discretion, in consultation with a health care practitioner, before undertaking the diet, exercise, and techniques described—particularly if you are having a high-risk pregnancy. The author and publisher expressly disclaim responsibility for any adverse effects that may result from the use or application of the information contained in this book.

All rights reserved, including the right to reproduce this book or portions thereof in any form whatsoever. For information, address Simon Element Subsidiary Rights Department, 1230 Avenue of the Americas, New York, NY 10020.

First Simon Element hardcover edition March 2026

SIMON ELEMENT and colophon are registered trademarks of Simon & Schuster, LLC

Simon & Schuster strongly believes in freedom of expression and stands against censorship in all its forms. For more information, visit BooksBelong.com.

For information about special discounts for bulk purchases, please contact Simon & Schuster Special Sales at 1-866-506-1949 or business@simonandschuster.com.

The Simon & Schuster Speakers Bureau can bring authors to your live event. For more information or to book an event, contact the Simon & Schuster Speakers Bureau at 1-866-248-3049 or visit our website at www.simonspeakers.com.

Recipe writer and food stylist: Annie Rigg
Recipe editor: Judy Barratt
Photography, design, and art direction: Smith & Gilmour
Props stylist: Hannah Wilkinson
Recipe Americanizer: Maria Zizka

Manufactured in the United States of America

1 3 5 7 9 10 8 6 4 2

Library of Congress Control Number has been applied for.

ISBN 978-1-6682-1912-6
ISBN 978-1-6682-1913-3 (ebook)

Let's stay in touch! Scan here to get book recommendations, exclusive offers, and more delivered to your inbox.

To all who mother—
in body, in spirit, in longing, or in memory.

Contents

You are not an oven 1

My story 10

The trimesters 17

Chapter 1 : The cookie equation 31

Chapter 2 : The six-egg problem 95

Chapter 3 : The real body-building 125

Chapter 4 : The underwater factor 173

Chapter 5 : The final crumbs 205

Giving birth 225

Breastfeeding and formula 246

Supplements 249

Trimester-by-trimester recap 253

All the best 262

Thank you 265

Scientific references 266

Index 267

Recipes 281

Dear reader, I've referred to the baby as "he" in this book, because I had a baby boy and I was thinking about him as I wrote. But please replace however you see fit.

You are not an oven

Have you ever baked something in an oven? A cake, a loaf of bread, vegetables? You set the oven's mode, its temperature, the timing, and your trusty appliance does what it promises: heats up the space to a number of degrees for a certain amount of time.

So let's say you are baking a delicious cake. You select, buy, measure, and prepare the ingredients. You sift them, melt them, whisk them, combine them. When the batter is done and you are satisfied with it, it goes into a pan, then into the oven in question. But importantly, once the cake is baking, it can no longer change. The oven can't transform a chocolate cake batter into an upside-down banana cake. It can't add sugar, tweak the amount of vanilla, or add more bananas. It can't change the quality of the flour or the provenance of the eggs. As long as it doesn't break on you, or randomly change its temperature along the way, the oven simply does its appointed job: it bakes. Everything else about the cake is already set.

With no transition, let's now talk about your *uterus*. Do you know what your uterus and the oven have in common? Not much. Even though you might have heard people say they have "a bun in the oven" when referring to growing a baby in their womb, this analogy is misleading: it implies that your baby is entirely predetermined when the sperm meets the egg. It sends the message that all you have to do now is keep the temperature at 98.6°F, try not to do anything obviously harmful (cigarettes, drugs, bungee-jumping while drinking vodka), and just wait forty or so weeks. It sends the message that you are a vessel of oxygen, nutrients, and heat, and that you are simply *allowing* your baby to grow. The conveyed sentiment is something along the lines of "don't stress, just let nature do its thing." But this is wrong.

My job is scientific research, and in my previous work I've explored how blood sugar affects our body and mind. I wrote two books in which I shared small habits that can keep our glucose levels steady to improve our health and well-being. It helped me, and lots of other people too. So when I became pregnant, I used those same skills. I dove into the latest studies on pregnancy nutrition conducted by scientists across the world. I found decades of published evidence, population surveys, and fantastic books—all full of crucial information that every mother needs to know. I found that we are far from simple ovens: during pregnancy, we are actively **influencing our baby**, his cognition, and his long-term health with what we eat—or don't eat—during these nine months.

I discovered many shocking facts—for example, that 90 percent of pregnant women are not eating enough choline, a key molecule (which we get from foods like animal liver and eggs) that forms a baby's brain cells in the womb, and that can positively influence his memory and attention levels. Seventy percent of us are also consuming too little protein, a lack that can not only erode our own muscle mass but may also program our baby's body to build less muscle and develop weaker organs. Other interesting research suggests that sugar cravings during pregnancy may be driven by an ancient biological mechanism—originally meant to ensure that we supplied enough energy for the baby—that's now backfiring in today's overly abundant food environment. Indeed, most of us eat more sugar when pregnant than when not pregnant (partly due to old wives' tales, such as "you're eating for two," which leads us to eat more sweet foods than we might need to). But sugar in pregnancy can impact your baby's brain development; and is linked to the likelihood of mental health disorders later in life, as well as diabetes, high blood pressure, and obesity as an adult. Worrying, to say the least. And gestational diabetes, a common condition during pregnancy in which your blood sugar levels become too high, also has a real impact on a baby's long-term health. Further, the majority of pregnant moms don't eat enough DHA during pregnancy. DHA is an omega-3 fatty acid that helps your baby's neurons (the brain cells that process information) connect with each other, while also lowering the risk of allergies and reducing the likelihood of preterm birth—a complication that is rising worldwide and carries its own long-term consequences. Along the way, I uncovered fascinating explanations for many common pregnancy experiences, from new insights into first-trimester nausea to how your body composition changes after birth.

I also learned something that changed the way I saw pregnancy forever: by the time your baby is born, the vast majority of his neurons are already formed—and *they won't get replaced*. This means the nutrients you provide during these nine months help shape the foundation of his brain for a lifetime.

Another key insight has to do with your baby's DNA. While you can't change the genetic code your baby inherits (half from the mom, half from the dad), the story doesn't end there. DNA is not a fixed script set in stone at conception. During pregnancy, something remarkable happens: **you influence which of your baby's genes are expressed and which remain silent.** This process, called epigenetics, works through chemical switches that turn genes on or off. Scientists call it **foetal programming**, and diet is one of the strongest forces shaping it. In practice, this means your baby is born with an epigenetic profile influenced by what you eat—and if you have multiple children and eat differently in your pregnancies, your children will be programmed differently.

The resounding message of all this research? That your diet while you are pregnant with your baby has a lifelong impact on him.

I know it's a lot to take in, and rest assured: it's not your fault that you don't know this. I didn't know any of it, either. If you've already had children, they are okay—your body has ways to compensate and ensure your baby grows in a healthy manner. But the power of nutrition is poorly communicated in standard medical care during pregnancy, and unless your job is to research scientific papers, the information is unlikely to just show up on your doorstep. What's more, the science is clear and exciting: diet during pregnancy plays a role in shaping your baby's development. It's *not* just a case of "set it and forget it," like a bun in the oven.

Indeed, another common but much more accurate way to describe the relationship between you and your baby is as a seed planted in soil. The seed contains crucial genetic instructions: whether it will become a palm tree, a rose bush, or a tomato vine. But as any good gardener knows (not me), the *soil* is crucial. It's not as simple as "plant it and it will grow tall and healthy." A rich, dense, diverse, fertilized soil will lead to a healthier tree than a soil that hasn't been tended to. The soil is co-creating the tree's genetic plan, and the tree will adapt to its environment, making do with less if less is available.

It's the same during pregnancy: your baby may not always get what he needs, and he will differ in who he is based on what he has access to and what he is exposed to in your womb. That gives you a lot more power than you have probably been told. While you can't choose the seed, you have an extraordinary influence over the soil.

When I first dove into the research, I was both shaken up and over-eager—cue swallowing chunks of frozen beef liver (more on that in Chapter 2). But I was also fascinated, and determined to put the most useful principles into practice. So I distilled everything into a handful of key habits that could improve my baby's health, and that I could actually manage while also crying constantly because of the hormones, juggling work, moving apartments, and feeling overwhelmed by all the planning to welcome my baby.

A few months later, I began sharing what I had learned with friends who were expecting. Their strong reactions to the science—first shock, then empowerment—made me realize just how deeply this information was needed. That's when I decided to gather it all into this book, so more people could benefit from it.

I've kept things simple: We start by looking at how diet affects your baby differently during the nausea-prone first trimester, compared to the rest of pregnancy. Then we dive into the heart of the book—**four chapters, each focused on a dietary principle designed to give your baby a powerful advantage for life, what I call the "pregnancy building blocks."** Every section is packed with cutting-edge science and concludes with an Action Plan providing practical tips and recommendations you can start using right away. Toward the end of the book, you'll find a final chapter on several smaller topics such as coffee and alcohol, then a deep dive into the science of labor and birth (as well as what helped me during them), guidance on breastfeeding and formula, a dedicated section on supplements, a full trimester-by-trimester recap, and the collection of scientific references. I end the book with recipes to help bring everything together.

Chapter 1 is all about what happens to your blood sugar during pregnancy. After you eat starches or sugars, your blood sugar (glucose) naturally rises. These increases are called glucose spikes. During pregnancy, your body becomes less efficient at handling them, so spikes can be sharper and last longer. This matters: they can program your baby's DNA toward certain outcomes, and even set the stage for a lifelong pull toward sugar. I'll also share what to do about cravings, and how managing sugar can lower your child's future risk of conditions like type 2 diabetes. In Chapter 2, you'll meet choline, an extraordinary nutrient hiding in plain sight, with a measurable influence on your baby's brain development. Chapter 3 will reframe how you think about protein, why your muscle mass matters during pregnancy, and why the fact that most of us are protein-restricted can impact our child's body composition even after birth. In Chapter 4, you'll discover DHA, an omega-3 fat derived from ocean algae that helps your baby's neurons connect and communicate, and which is essential for brain wiring in the womb. Most moms are not getting enough of these three building blocks—choline, protein, and DHA. In fact, **studies show fewer than 10 percent of pregnant women in high-income countries reach optimal levels**. Like I say, this isn't (yet) common knowledge.

I'll end the introduction with this: when you are pregnant, you are a scientist-magician-life-grower with real superpowers. And if you know how to use them, you can positively impact your baby's health for his entire life. So let's get to it.

Some quick housekeeping

First things first: if you don't do any of the things in this book, your child will most likely turn out fine. When my mother was pregnant with me, she ate Special K cereal with a mountain of sugar on top every morning for breakfast—and washed it down with Diet Coke. And I ended up okay: aside from an unhealthy obsession with cats and a daily existential crisis or two—totally normal.

Except . . . in all fairness, there's a long list of physical and mental health issues I've experienced over the years, from panic attacks and depersonalization (a condition with which you feel like a stranger in your own body), to borderline prediabetes in my twenties. And I can't help but wonder: *What if some of them trace back to what was happening in the womb?* Maybe it was the Diet Coke, maybe it was fate, maybe I was just destined to be a cat enthusiast with mild existential dread. I'll never know for sure—and actually nor do I need to: I'm a functioning, mostly healthy adult, and I get along fine.

So if you've had kids before and were not aware of this science, or if you're only discovering this book late in pregnancy, don't worry. When it comes to the fundamentals of growing a baby, you already have them: your body (including your uterus) and access to oxygen and food.

While the science in this book may seem overwhelming at first, it's certainly not intended to make you feel guilty or scared. It's here if you're curious about the extra optimizations you can make. Even if you take just a few ideas from these pages and use them now and then, that's fantastic. You don't have to do everything every day (I certainly didn't manage to).

I should also add that this science is by no means a magic bullet to the perfect pregnancy and the perfectly healthy baby. You could follow every principle in this book to the letter and still face things that are beyond your control (I'll share a recent experience of my own on the following pages). What you eat is not the only factor shaping your baby's health: access to medical care, socio-economic status, the environment your baby is born into, genetics, sheer luck or randomness, things that we don't understand yet, and more, play their part too.

Pregnancy may be a time when you feel like many of the changes that are happening to your body are out of your control, but nutrition is one of the few things you *can* influence—and the simple, science-backed changes I am proposing can genuinely give your baby a stronger start. Today, with chronic diseases on the rise and ever-younger people facing challenges like mental health disorders, diabetes, and high blood pressure, anything that strengthens the womb environment matters—especially given the amount of research pointing to links between a baby's experience in utero and the risk of these, as you'll soon learn. The point is: if you are in the know, you might as well put as many odds in your baby's favor as you can. And you don't need to wait until you get pregnant—applying the principles in this book prepregnancy will help set you up for success. It's never too early to start.

Second bit of housekeeping: I'm a biochemist, not a doctor. Think of me like a science translator or teacher. I gather published research from scientists around the world, health agency guidelines, physiology textbooks, and break them down into simple, practical insights you can actually use. As a result, everything in these pages is based on population-level data and guidelines—it's meant to inform and empower, not to diagnose, cure, prevent, or treat any condition or disease. It doesn't account for your unique medical history or circumstances, and isn't medical advice, so it's essential to check with your care team and a qualified provider before making any changes to how you eat or manage your health.

My story

Trigger warning: this section discusses pregnancy loss. If that's not something you want to read about today, go straight to the next chapter.

Dear reader: if we haven't met yet, I'm Jessie. It's nice to meet you. I wrote most of this book while I was pregnant with my first-born, a son. But this wasn't my first pregnancy. I want to share the story of what happened, because I felt so alone when it did and I wished more people had shared their own journey with me.

I first became pregnant at 31 years old, two months after removing my IUD. My husband and I were really happy that it happened so quickly. I told everyone straightaway (literally the day I got the positive pregnancy test), and I started preparing myself for the fact that our baby would be born in December.

I began researching pregnancy nutrition, and started writing the first few pages of this book. I went into my scans with great enthusiasm: it didn't even cross my mind that something could go wrong. The health of the baby wasn't a concern—I was, however, stressed about all the usual things: where I was going to give birth, whether we needed to move apartments . . . It all felt very real, very fast. I had my first scan at just five weeks—we could see a tiny little amorphous thing. Then our second scan a month later, around ten weeks: we heard the heartbeat and we saw the embryo, a bit less tiny, little amorphous thing. It was a great experience.

Even though I started getting quite nauseous around that time, we still felt very excited, picking out names, and wondering about the baby's sex. At around 14 weeks, we were back in the doctor's office for our next routine check. And, as usual, I lay back on the table and the doctor put some gel on my lower stomach and I watched the screen for the image to come up. As soon as it appeared, I knew the pregnancy was over—the little embryo hadn't changed much since the previous time, and it was at the bottom of my uterus, scrunched up and lifeless, like you would imagine a dead fish at the bottom of an aquarium.

After ten seconds of silence the doctor confirmed what I had already understood: there was no more heartbeat. The pregnancy had stopped a full three weeks previously (around 10½ weeks), and I hadn't even known. I hadn't felt anything, nor had any miscarriage symptoms. It's called a "silent" miscarriage. The embryo stops developing, dies, but your body does not expel it.

I felt like life had been knocked out of me. I started sobbing as the doctor told me that I needed to have a procedure. I was in complete and utter shock—from thinking I would be a mom in six months, I now had to accept that it was all over. Legs-stop-working-drop-to-the-ground sort of pain. I remember later screaming in my living room and begging the universe for my baby back. Arguing that the doctor must be wrong and that he had made a mistake. I was really confused about my relationship with my body—that the dead embryo had been inside me for almost a month and I had known nothing about it; and that I now had to live with it still there, until the procedure. I couldn't believe this had happened.

I think one of the reasons I was in so much shock and disbelief is that the idea of a miscarriage was not really in my consciousness.

Yes, I had friends going through IVF who had experienced one, but I didn't know that miscarriage is also common in people who are trying to conceive naturally. I wasn't prepared for the possibility, partly, I suppose, because it is rarely discussed. I thought: "I'm young, I'm healthy, what can go wrong?" I didn't know that miscarriages can happen to anyone: that about one in five pregnancies end this way. And even though I subsequently learned that my pregnancy loss was probably due to DNA abnormalities beyond my control, I of course wondered if it was something I did.

So we found a hospital, and when they informed me that I would need to go under general anaesthesia for the procedure (a vacuum aspiration) that was even harder to deal with. I hate going under: it reminds me of a traumatic spine surgery I went through when I was 19 years old.

As I conveyed the sad news to the people around me, the reactions ranged from helpful and supportive, to very out-of-touch—"don't think about it." To feel less lonely, I looked up "celebrities who have had miscarriages." It sounds silly, but I desperately wanted to feel some sense of kinship, connection. I wanted to know that other people had gone through this too. The more I reached out, the more tongues untied and I learned that many people close to me had also had the experience of pregnancy loss—but they had never mentioned it before. This seemed tragic to me. I felt desolate, and an utter wreck.

The procedure was scheduled to take place on a Friday at 1 p.m. The night before it, I had been invited to go on one of the biggest evening live TV shows in France, something I had been really looking forward to. I could have canceled at this point, but I didn't. From a career perspective, it was one of the most important weeks ever for me; from a personal perspective, one of the worst in my life. As I walked onto the set and pretended everything was absolutely fantastic, (3 ... 2 ... 1 ... *you're live*), I did my best to hold it together—to manage the idea of the dead embryo in my womb while doing my work justice on this show.

Then came the procedure. I kept repeating to myself something that a close friend had said to me: "May this passing be peaceful." This sentence still makes me cry. I woke up from the anesthesia. I felt really sad, really mad, and so empty.

It was June. A week later it was my birthday. By now, my despair had turned into anger: Why do some people have pregnancies where everything is fine—where they're not stressed, they have no issues—and I have to go through this? It was hard to process. Unimaginable gut-wrenching pain and having to hold back tears every time I saw a pregnant woman on the street.

The hormones dropping away combined with the grief put me in a frantic spiral for weeks as I experienced every single emotion at once. I had to rewire my brain, my expectations, our timeline. I also felt embarrassed and ashamed. People do not know how to talk about pregnancy loss. I felt that I made those around me uncomfortable. I oscillated between thinking "Why is nobody asking me how I'm doing?" to "I hope no one mentions it." So then on top of being mad at the world, I was mad at my family and my friends for not knowing how to handle it. Great.

I drank inordinate quantities of coffee and numbed myself with work. Writing helped, singing helped, speaking to people who had gone through this and were able to talk about it openly helped. Reading other people's stories helped. My husband just being there helped. What *didn't* help was seeing people announcing their pregnancies online ("Why is everyone having a baby all of a sudden?").

And then I got the all-clear from the doctor. At first, I thought I needed to be completely emotionally healed from the pregnancy loss before it was okay to try again. I quickly understood that this would never happen. The grief of the loss would always be there, coexisting with whatever else happened in my life. So we started trying again, and it was really difficult. The uncertainty, the wondering if it would take years, the many, many pregnancy tests, the hope, the stress. It was a real trial of the heart.

I was still grieving three months later when I got a positive pregnancy test again. I knew I was really lucky that it had happened so quickly. But I couldn't square in my mind the happy news with the grief I still felt. So I didn't allow myself to be happy. I didn't allow myself to even believe in this pregnancy. I was 100 percent certain I was going to miscarry again. We didn't tell anyone. We didn't get emotionally attached at all. It felt too vulnerable to do so.

I had a very challenging first trimester, not because of the nausea—which was easier this time—but because of the constant, crippling anxiety, the checking of my underwear for blood every time I went to the bathroom, the daily internet rabbit holes ("If I feel nauseous one day and then the next day not, does it mean I have had a silent miscarriage?"), the crying, the stress (and the doctor urging me *not* to stress—so helpful, thanks).

I sobbed for 24 hours before each scan, fearing I would again see a lifeless little embryo on the screen. Each time, as I was given good news—"everything is fine"/"the blood test is normal"/"it's going well, see you in a month"—I was happy for 48 hours. Then the anxiety and fear would creep back in. I wished I could have an ultrasound every day to put my mind at ease. At three months I tried to shift my feelings about it all. I wanted to allow myself to believe in this baby, instead of being constantly convinced the worst would happen. My therapist said something beautiful that really helped: "You don't know what is going to happen. But you can allow yourself to love this baby for as long as he is with you." I slowly opened my heart to some joy—the first time I felt him kick was wonderful . . . But then I didn't feel anything for two weeks. Cue anxiety all over again.

About five months into the pregnancy, I started to breathe easier. I felt like things might turn out okay. The daily kicks really helped. We told our friends around this time. I started writing this book again.

I'm sharing all this because, while I consider myself pretty well informed, I was absolutely not prepared for this miscarriage. It hit me hard. I hope things will change—that pregnancy loss will become less of a taboo, and that we will all become better equipped to support people going through it. And, in case this has also happened to you and you felt alone too, I hope that sharing this story was a little bit helpful.

The experience of losing my first pregnancy profoundly changed me. It made me deeply appreciate how precious and fragile the process of creating a life can be. Because yes, there is so much we can't control—how long it takes us to conceive, how we feel along the way, whether loss happens. But there are also things we *can* control. And one of the most powerful is what we put on our plate during the crucial nine months of pregnancy—how we nourish our body and our baby, day by day. Through the choices we make about food, we hold quiet superpowers. These are opportunities like no other. That's what this book is about.

The trimesters

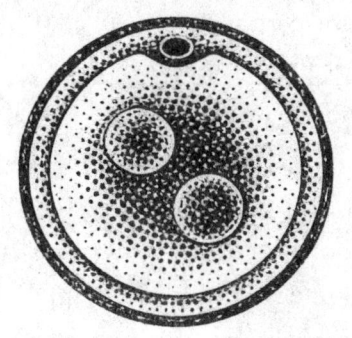

Picture this: You wake up in the middle of the night. Your room is pitch-black. You need to find something you left somewhere in your apartment—but you're not allowed to turn on the lights. You get up, bump into furniture, fumble your way around. Not easy, right?

That's basically what it's like to be a tiny sperm in the fallopian tube: completely blind, swimming upstream through cervical and uterine fluids, all while dodging attacks from the woman's immune system, which treats sperm like intruders. Out of the millions released during sex, only about 250 make it anywhere near the egg. And this is where the egg takes charge—releasing a chemical "scent" that acts like a beacon to guide sperm toward it. Even more fascinating, that scent seems to be selective: the egg may actually draw in certain sperm over others, perhaps those that are most genetically compatible.

Once chosen and allowed to enter, the sperm's head penetrates the membrane of the egg. Almost immediately, microscopic helpers carried by the egg, called enzymes, spring into action in order to do something rather harsh: *digest* the sperm's head membrane to release the DNA trapped inside. In essence, the sperm's head *explodes*, pouring out its genetic material. Intense, but necessary.

One thing that makes the sperm's quest a little easier is the sheer size of the egg. If a sperm were the size of a grain of rice, the egg beside it would be a basketball—nearly 10,000 times larger. Why the difference? Because sperm travel light: their only job is to deliver half the genetic code. The egg, by contrast, comes fully stocked with *food*, nutrients, and raw materials to sustain the first five to seven days of development.

Once the sperm and the egg fuse, the newly formed single

cell containing a full set of genes will start to divide. Within 24 hours, it will become two cells. And in the next 12 hours or so, these two cells will become four.

The first week of embryonic development

| EGG | FERTILIZATION 12 to 24h | SINGLE CELL 24h | FIRST DIVISION 24h |

| 2-CELL STAGE 36h | 4-CELL STAGE 48h | 100 CELLS 5 days | 500+ CELLS 9 days |

For the first few days of development, the egg provides the necessary supplies to support cell division.

Over the next nine months, these cells will continue to divide and multiply to drive the development of your baby, as well as that of the placenta, an important temporary organ you will learn about soon. If there are no bumps in the road (DNA abnormalities, or many other potential issues), the newly formed embryo will comprise about 100 cells at day five, one *million* cells three weeks post-conception, and just over one *trillion* cells at birth. That's a whole lot of cells to make.

The first trimester: nausea and chocolate croissants

So how exactly do these one trillion cells that will form your baby come to be in your uterus? "Nothing is lost, nothing is created, everything is transformed," famously stated Antoine Lavoisier, a French chemist often referred to as the Father of Modern Chemistry. The materials that compose these cells, that compose your baby, don't come out of thin air: they must come from somewhere . . . and that somewhere is you. After the first five days, when the food in the egg has been used up to make the first 100 cells, your embryo shifts to a much larger source of nutrition: to make the remaining 999,999,999,900 cells, it relies purely on nutrients you have stored in your body and on the food you will eat during the pregnancy.

In the first trimester, your embryo is not yet connected to your bloodstream. Instead, growth depends on a kind of "uterine milk," a fluid secreted by glands in the lining of your uterus, which contains everything the early cells need to develop. Supporting the process is the yolk sac—a small but mighty structure that sits just outside the embryo, transferring nutrients from the uterine secretions and even producing your baby's very first blood cells.

At this stage, having good nutrient reserves and taking the right supplements can help the uterine glands do their job. However, it's different from the second and third trimesters, when your bloodstream and your baby's are directly connected through the placenta, as we'll see.

This can be a comforting thought for the 60 to 90 percent of women who experience nausea in early pregnancy and find their diets suddenly . . . less than ideal. It happened to me too, despite my own confidence that I would dodge it. My mom had told me she never felt sick during her pregnancies, so naturally I assumed I'd inherited her symptom-free experience. In week seven, woken up in the middle of the night by an uncontrollable urge to throw up, I was proved very wrong. Humility: 1. Jessie: 0.

Lo and behold, for a good chunk of my second, third, and even a bit of my fourth month of pregnancy, I was nauseous. On those days, my diet revolved almost entirely around pastries and pasta. Occasionally, I could manage some yogurt, a handful of nuts, and—every few days, if I was lucky—a piece of fish or meat in the evening (as long as there were chips right there too). But truly, carbs were the only thing that made the nausea back off. So I ate a lot of carbs. I still remember near the end of the third month, the day I suddenly thought: "I think I could eat an avocado." Something *green*! This was a big moment.

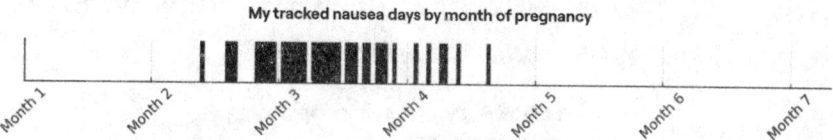

My nausea days during pregnancy, tracked from the day of my last period before conception. Nausea generally shows up between the 4th and 7th week, and goes away by the second trimester, but every pregnancy is very different.

For decades, scientists believed that what made mothers-to-be nauseous was a hormone called hCG. This hormone is produced in your uterus by the cells that will develop into the placenta. It increases significantly during the beginning of pregnancy and tells your body to keep your uterus intact (instead of shedding its lining and having a period). It's the hormone that a pregnancy test detects in your pee to tell you if you're pregnant. And it all seemed to make perfect sense, because if you track the level of hCG during the first few months of pregnancy, it correlates quite well to when nausea develops, peaks, and drops. In a recent study looking at data tracked from close to 200,000 pregnant women, the prevalence of nausea was as follows:

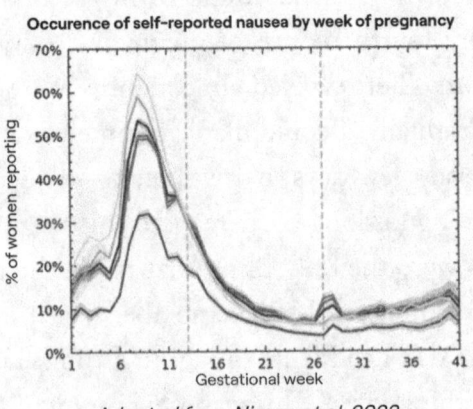

Adapted from Nissen et al. 2023

And hCG levels per week, as determined on around 8,000 women, look approximately the same:

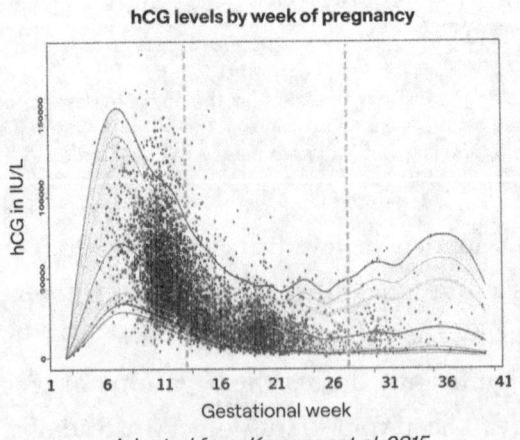

Adapted from Korevaar et al. 2015

Yet recent studies are shifting away from the idea that hCG causes nausea. This is because hCG levels have not been found to be significantly different between women with and without hyperemesis gravidarum, an extreme type of pregnancy nausea. Instead, scientists have found that the cause might be a hormone **produced by the placenta and the fetus** called GDF15. And that whether or not we get nauseous may be more dependent on the level of GDF15 we had in our body before and how it compares to our levels during pregnancy.

While this is interesting, I'm sorry to say that this new discovery isn't all that helpful if you're experiencing nausea. But here are some tips for what to do about it.

✴ NAUSEA TIPS ✴

✴ If you can, eat some protein first thing in the morning before moving around too much, as protein tends to help reduce nausea. Proteins include animal foods like eggs, meat, fish, dairy (Greek yogurt worked pretty well for me—try it out), and nuts or seeds (I would keep almonds on my nightstand and have a handful before getting out of bed).

✴ Invest in some very strong ginger nausea gummies (head to www.glucosegoddess.com/pages/best-ginger-gummies or scan the QR code for which ones I recommend).

Nausea gummies

* Avoid blood sugar crashes. (In Chapter 1, we go into blood sugar in detail.) This is because low blood sugar levels are common in early pregnancy and one of their side effects can be an exacerbation of nausea. Some scientists have proposed that overnight fasting reduces glucose levels, and that low glucose in the morning could trigger nausea. Here again, eating protein first thing can help, as can eating lots of small meals containing some amount of carbs throughout the day, rather than a lot of carbs all at once.

* Add clothing to your carbs. If you can, as you eat your carbs throughout the day, pair them with some protein, fat, or fiber. Not only will this stabilize your blood sugar, it's also a good way to get some nutrition in. For example, if you're going to have a piece of toast, add some (pasteurized) goat cheese to it. Or, add a bit of olive oil to some pasta, and maybe throw in a handful of spinach leaves. Or, when you eat a cookie, pair it with a few spoonfuls of Greek yogurt.

* Rely on lots of snacks. As I mentioned above, eating little and often usually helps nausea—the key here is to snack on things that will not start a blood sugar roller coaster. Not only would I eat almonds before getting out of bed, I kept a packet in my handbag and would eat them throughout the day. Other examples: a yogurt, a cracker with a piece of cheese, an apple with nut butter, berries, seaweed snacks, or a slice of toast with some butter or cream cheese.

* If your nausea subsides during the day, take advantage of the release to eat something nutritious: again, Greek yogurt is

a great move, or some grilled chicken, eggs, or fruit with nut butter. If you can do this once or twice a week even, that's great.

✳ Choose starches over sugars. We will cover *why* in Chapter 1, but if you can choose between something starchy (bread, pasta, rice, potatoes, oats) and something sweet (like a cake, cookie, or dessert), the starchy option is a better choice for your body. That's because starches don't contain fructose, but sugars do, and fructose is harmful for our bodies in large quantities.

✳ My last tip is not evidence-based but I found that several times when I ate meat at night, my nausea was a bit better in the morning. Maybe something to do with the protein—I don't know—but it might work for you.

First-trimester nausea made me feel bloated and quite rubbish. While it would of course be ideal to have a great diet during this time too, it's just not realistic for most of us. Throw any guilt out the window and just do what you can. If it's helpful, picture me eating pains au chocolat three times a day for breakfast, lunch, and dinner. It's okay, your baby is okay. For most women, things will get better in the second and third trimesters and, with the science you'll learn in this book, you'll be set up for feeling amazing.

At the end of the first trimester (around weeks 10–12), when the placenta becomes fully functional and your baby becomes connected to your bloodstream, most women find their nausea lessens and then disappears. I was still nauseous for another month or so, so I didn't hit full stride in terms of my nutrition goals until week 14-ish, but things were looking up. In any case, the second trimester is the turning point: this is when things start to get interesting.

The second and third trimesters: welcome to the placenta

The placenta is a remarkable, temporary organ that you grow next to your baby, inside your uterus, and that you deliver after the birth. If you have multiple pregnancies, you will grow a whole new one for each baby. Its role is to feed your baby by connecting your blood supply to your baby's bloodstream, via the uterine wall on one side and the umbilical cord on the other. For the remaining two trimesters of pregnancy, all the nutrition your baby receives will come from your bloodstream through the placenta.

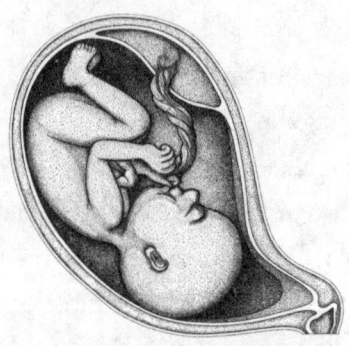

The placenta attaches to the inside of your uterus, connecting to your bloodstream on one side and leading to your baby's umbilical cord and circulation on the other.

Leonardo da Vinci was among the first to study and sketch the placenta in detail around 1510. He understood that this organ was very important to the fetus, but mistakenly concluded that the mother's blood and the baby's blood mixed together inside it. This idea persisted until the 19th century when scientists began to realize that instead of being a mixing bowl, the placenta might act as a filter.

By the 1920s, the work of researchers using advanced microscopes discovered the truth: the mother's and baby's blood never mix. Instead, the placenta contains a specialized membrane that brings the two bloodstreams into *very* close contact in order for nutrients, oxygen, and waste to pass from one to the other—without ever combining them.

What does the placenta do, exactly? The common belief that "your baby will get what it needs from you" suggests that the placenta carefully selects what passes through, letting in only the good while keeping out the bad. But the reality is quite different. The placenta isn't a strict bouncer at a nightclub, deciding who gets in and who doesn't. Instead, this organ is more akin to a manager following broad guidelines: *"Let anyone in who is under six feet tall, and as long as there are more people in line outside than inside the club, keep bringing people in."* Rather than making conscious choices, the placenta follows biological rules based on molecule size and concentration. Anything in high concentration in your bloodstream will naturally diffuse into your baby's blood—as long as it's small enough to cross the membrane (some things are too big, for example red blood cells and molecules such as insulin—more on that shortly). This process works in much the same way that a smell diffuses through a room, moving from areas of high concentration to low concentration.

This is why if you drink alcohol, take drugs, or ingest or inhale toxins such as cigarette smoke, these substances will arrive in your baby's blood, even though they aren't helpful. Basically, **the placenta largely "trusts" that whatever is in your blood belongs in your baby's blood**. So what you eat will directly be reflected in your baby's blood composition. This may sound like quite a daunting responsibility, because, yes, in some cases, too much of a substance from food can have negative consequences; but looked at another way, it actually gives you more power than you have probably been told. Every positive choice you make is a positive choice for your child too—like eating the foods you'll learn about in this book.

For your unborn baby, much is happening. He is now going to be impacted every minute of every day by the nutrients coming through the placenta. Whereas in the first trimester, he was fed through uterine milk, now your bloodstreams are almost one. He is connected to you and to the variations of nutrients in your blood. A symbiosis is established.

This process is, once again, akin to how a seed grows into a tree. The seed itself contains reserves for the first few days of growth. Then it starts to grow roots—just like when your baby shifts from being nourished by egg reserves and uterine milk to being fed through the placenta and umbilical cord. The tree's roots burrow into the soil, ideally pulling from it what it *needs*, but more often than not, simply what it *can*. Depending on the soil (and the sunlight and the air), the tree will grow strong and healthy, or less strong and less healthy.

In the same way, one of the biggest misconceptions about pregnancy is that your baby will take *everything he needs* from you, and he will always have access to the perfect amount of nourishment he requires to thrive. The reality is that once the placenta is in place, your baby will take what he *can*, depending on what is available. He can't communicate with you, but he's in there hoping you will give him all the best stuff.

And as I explained in the introduction, what you eat throughout the trimesters will influence your baby's body, brain, and future health risk. As a pregnant mother-to-be, you are currently in a position to shape your child's life in a profound way. Every single one of his trillion cells are forming right there, with great sensitivity to the environment in your womb, and the quantities of nutrients you make available will impact his future.

You aren't just an oven. So it's time to get to our first concept.

CHAPTER 1

The cookie equation

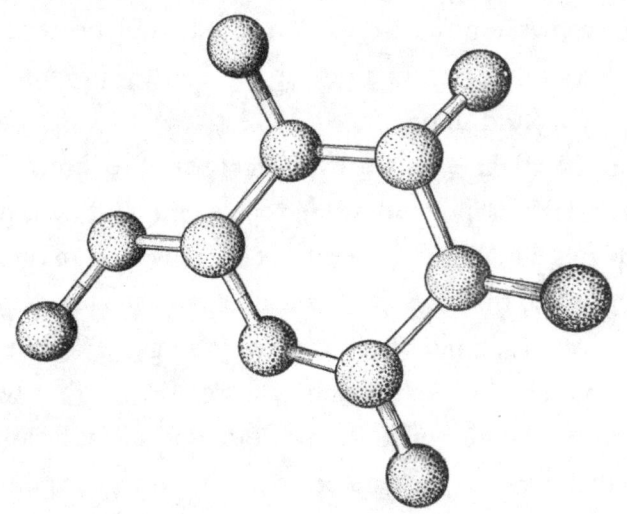

GLUCOSE

While you were reading the previous section on the three trimesters, if you were reading at an average speed, you took around 200 breaths. Do you know why you breathe? To supply your body with something essential: oxygen from the air. With each of the 20,000 breaths you take daily, countless oxygen molecules flow from your nose to your lungs, where they get transferred to your bloodstream, then pumped throughout your body by your heart. And oxygen's job? To get to your **mitochondria**: the microscopic energy factories housed in each of your trillions of cells. As energy factories, these mitochondria use the oxygen you just inhaled to create, well, *energy*. The technical name for this energy is adenosine triphosphate, or ATP, and it is required by every organ in your body to perform its function: your brain needs ATP to think, your heart to pump, your muscles to walk, your stomach to digest, your lymph nodes to protect you, and so on.

During pregnancy, your baby doesn't yet have direct access to air as he is floating in liquid inside your uterus. But he is perfectly fine with this situation. *You* are the one delivering oxygen to his mitochondria so that they can make energy to create organs, form brain connections, build bones, and everything else. While you are carrying your child in your womb, you are breathing for two.

In an amazing demonstration of biological adaptation, pregnancy transforms the way you breathe without you even realizing it. Over these nine months, hormones gently reprogram your lungs, not to increase how many breaths you take, but to make each of them 30 to 50 percent deeper by the third trimester. With every deeper inhale, you're drawing in significantly more oxygen, sending it coursing through your bloodstream to fuel both your body and your growing baby.

Glucose, we meet again

Along with oxygen, the other essential substance that mitochondria need in order to produce energy is glucose. While oxygen comes from the air we breathe, glucose comes from the food we eat. Glucose is present in foods called "carbohydrates," or "carbs" for short, which include both **starches** (bread, pasta, flour, rice, potatoes, oats . . .) and **sugars** (anything sweet, from a banana to chocolate ice cream). When we eat starches or sugars, our digestive system breaks them down into glucose, which then enters our bloodstream. We will cover other nutrients such as proteins, fats, fiber, vitamins, and minerals in more detail in later parts of the book. But for now, let's focus on glucose.

Glucose is crucial to human life. Once it is in our bloodstream, it rushes through our body and gets used by our mitochondria, along with oxygen, to create energy. Glucose is so essential to our body's energy-producing activity that if we don't eat any, our liver will create it from within.

Giving our body *some* glucose through eating carbs is great. But *too much* glucose is bad news. I wrote an entire book about this, called *Glucose Revolution*, but the main idea is simple: too much glucose—from a diet very high in starches and sugars—causes problems. It's like giving too much water to a plant: water is essential in the right amount, yet an excess drowns the roots.

While we used to believe that managing glucose levels mattered only for those with a diabetes diagnosis, now we understand it's paramount for all—including, as we shall soon discover, for a developing baby.

Picture your last meal: if it had carbohydrates in it, those carbs will have turned to glucose during digestion, then entered your bloodstream by diffusing through your gut lining. The concentration of glucose in your bloodstream, also referred to as your "blood sugar levels," will have increased.

Let's take two examples to show you how it works: if your meal was composed of only carbs, such as a plate of pasta (starch), with bread (starch), a fruit juice (sugar), and a cookie (starch and sugar), those foods will all have turned to glucose as you digested them, and your blood sugar levels will have skyrocketed for a couple of hours. This sharp rise in the concentration of glucose in your bloodstream is called a glucose *spike*. If, on the other hand, you ate a meal containing *some* carbs, for example rice (starch), but other foods too—such as fish (protein), avocado (fat), asparagus (fiber), and Greek yogurt (fat and protein, a tiny bit of natural milk sugar)—your glucose will have risen more moderately.

In the images below you can see my glucose levels as measured by a continuous glucose monitor, a small device I wore that measured my glucose around the clock and sent the data straight to my phone.

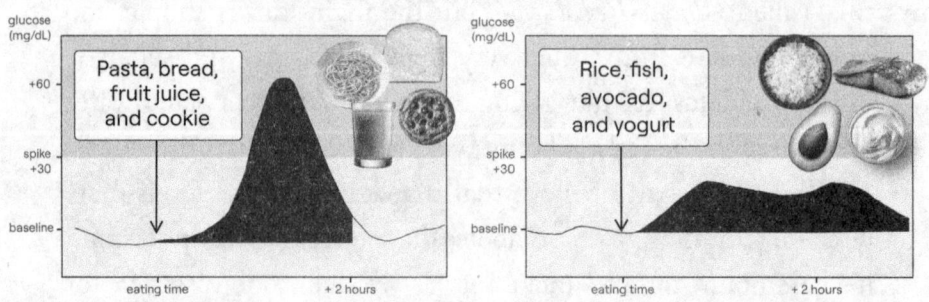

The glucose increase in my body after eating a meal high in carbs (left graph) compared to a meal lower in carbs (right graph).

For a handy reference, in the Action Plan at the end of this chapter (see pages 71–93) I've included a table that shows which foods turn to glucose during digestion and which don't.

Moderate fluctuations in glucose levels, such as the one from the balanced meal with rice, fish, avocado, and yogurt in the graphs, are completely normal. But spiking our glucose levels very high and frequently, as is unfortunately the case for many of us today because our modern diets are very high in carbs and sugars, leads to unwanted consequences.

The first of these consequences is **inflammation**. Your mitochondria love a steady supply of glucose to use to make energy, but having to deal with big glucose spikes renders them overwhelmed and stressed. And this in turn increases inflammation in your body. Some inflammation is normal—it's your body's defense mechanism against invaders, or pathogens. But chronic inflammation is the constant, dysregulated, and problematic activity of your immune system against your own body. And it's no joke—today, **three out of five people will die from an inflammation-based condition**, including heart disease, stroke, and diabetes.

The second consequence of large glucose spikes is **insulin release**. When your body detects excess glucose arriving from, say, a spaghetti-and-chocolate-cake meal, your pancreas releases a hormone called **insulin** to clear it out. Insulin works like an usher that directs excess glucose to various storage units in your body so that it doesn't stay at high levels in your bloodstream for too long (as that will increase inflammation). It grabs the excess glucose and stows it away, first in your liver, then in your muscles. When both of these places are full, any remaining excess glucose gets converted to fat and stored in your *fat cells*. This is one of the ways that you grow **fat mass in your body**.

Incidentally, as I alluded to earlier, starches and sugars are not equal in this game of consequences. Sugars increase inflammation and fat storage more than starches do. This is because, while starches contain only glucose, sugars contain glucose *and fructose*, another molecule that has more damaging consequences than glucose alone. So sugars create a glucose spike and a fructose spike too. If you're choosing between bread (starch) or a cake (which contains sugar), the bread will be better for your body—and as you will see, also for your developing baby. (A note on fruit: although whole fruit contains sugar, aka glucose and fructose, it does not affect you in the same way because of the protective action of the fiber the fruit contains. Fiber slows down the absorption of glucose and fructose. If, however, you juice, blend, or purée whole fruit, there will be no intact fiber left to protect you, and the fructose will have a detrimental impact.)

One last thing on glucose spikes. They have a cumulative impact on your **fasting** glucose level. This is your "baseline" glucose level, measured by the concentration of glucose in your blood first thing in the morning after you have fasted overnight. The more glucose spikes you experience throughout your life, the more insulin gets released, the more your storage units fill up. But with a limit: eventually, they become full, and excess glucose has nowhere to go so your baseline glucose level rises. When you aren't pregnant, your fasting glucose levels are considered normal up to 100mg/dL (above 100mg/dL, you are diagnosed with prediabetes, and above 126mg/dL, with type 2 diabetes). Yet lower is likely better: recent studies are showing that keeping glucose levels around 85mg/dL may actually be ideal.

During pregnancy, however, a few things change with regards to your blood sugar. And that's what we are going to look at next.

The nine-month glucose shift

When you are pregnant, your fasting, or "baseline," glucose level naturally runs lower. There are a few theories as to why this happens—for example, because of hormonal changes, or as the biological result of your placenta and your baby continuously pulling from your glucose levels for their own needs. It's also the result of a dilution effect: your blood volume during pregnancy increases by about 50 percent, going from 2.6 liters to roughly 3.8 liters. With a higher volume of blood, the concentration of glucose in it reduces slightly.

Now, because glucose levels naturally run lower during pregnancy, instead of the "healthy" range being considered anything below 100mg/dL, the "healthy" range when you are pregnant is considered to be anything below 92mg/dL. When I was pregnant, I tested my fasting glucose levels regularly with blood draws: they usually sat around 79mg/dL, compared to 87mg/dL when not pregnant.

That's glucose. Now, to insulin—the hormone in charge of putting glucose away after you eat. As we saw, insulin acts like an usher: it unlocks your liver, muscle, and fat cells to let glucose in, so that it can be stored away and bring your blood sugar levels back down.

During pregnancy, insulin still has this job. But there's one important change: your cells become less responsive to it. The "locks" on those storage doors get harder to open. This means insulin isn't as effective at clearing glucose after meals. We describe this as the body becoming *more resistant to* insulin—a normal and expected shift during pregnancy.

As a result, after you eat, glucose from your food stays elevated in the bloodstream for longer than it normally would. It does eventually come back down, but it takes more time.

This insulin resistance gradually increases throughout pregnancy, becoming more pronounced as you near your due date. For example: if you eat a cookie in your first trimester, your glucose spike (the rise and fall in blood glucose after you eat it) might look similar to how it would have looked before pregnancy. However, from around 20 weeks (4½ months) onward, your glucose will increase more after eating the same food, and stay elevated for longer before returning to baseline.

In the graphs opposite, you'll see a month-by-month visual of how the same cookie causes bigger and longer spikes as pregnancy progresses because of the increase in insulin resistance.

Increased insulin resistance during pregnancy is not random: your body does this purposely. And there's one main theory to explain it: after eating, your body is focused on keeping glucose around in the bloodstream so that your placenta and your baby have access to more of it. Just as your own cells rely on glucose for energy, your placenta and your growing baby also have cells hungry for glucose. With more glucose hanging around in your bloodstream rather than being quickly ushered away, it gives more time for your developing baby and the placenta to pull from it.

From an evolutionary perspective, this strategy makes a lot of sense. In a world before supermarkets, where glucose was hard to come by—found mostly in seasonal fruits or starchy roots—keeping a generous amount of glucose in the bloodstream helped ensure that a growing baby got enough fuel, even when food was scarce. But today, with modern diets overloaded with refined sugars and starches, this ancient biological adaptation can backfire. Our body's pregnancy responses haven't changed—but our food has.

With its increased insulin resistance, our system is primed to make the most of what it gets—to extract more "value" from even small amounts of glucose by keeping it in our bloodstream

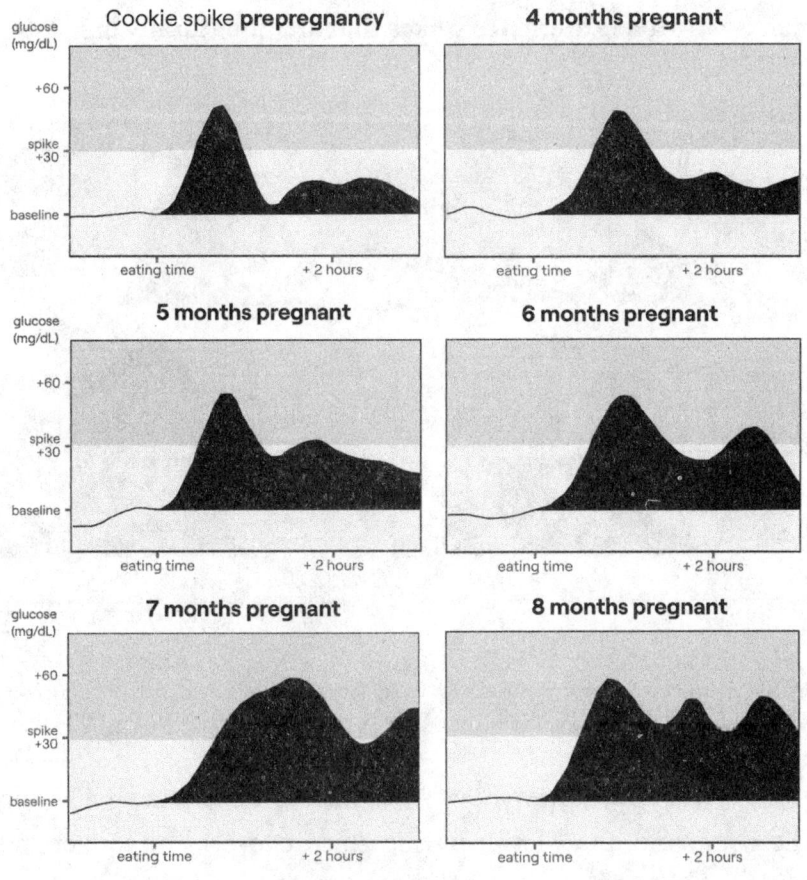

The glucose spike from a cookie, prepregnancy, at month 4, 5, 6, 7, and 8. The same cookie is causing bigger and longer spikes as pregnancy progresses because of an increase in insulin resistance. The "waves" you see on the spikes reflect insulin's successive attempts to bring glucose back down, but you can ignore them and look at the big picture: higher and longer spikes as the months pass.

for longer. We really don't need to eat more starches and sugar when we're pregnant. Tiny amounts already go a long way.

In my ninth month of pregnancy, I was shocked by what I saw on my glucose monitor—there was a huge difference compared to my glucose spikes before pregnancy (see graphs below). The takeaway here: our biological adaptation is no match for our modern, sugar-filled diet, and as a consequence during pregnancy **we often experience spikes that are unnaturally big**.

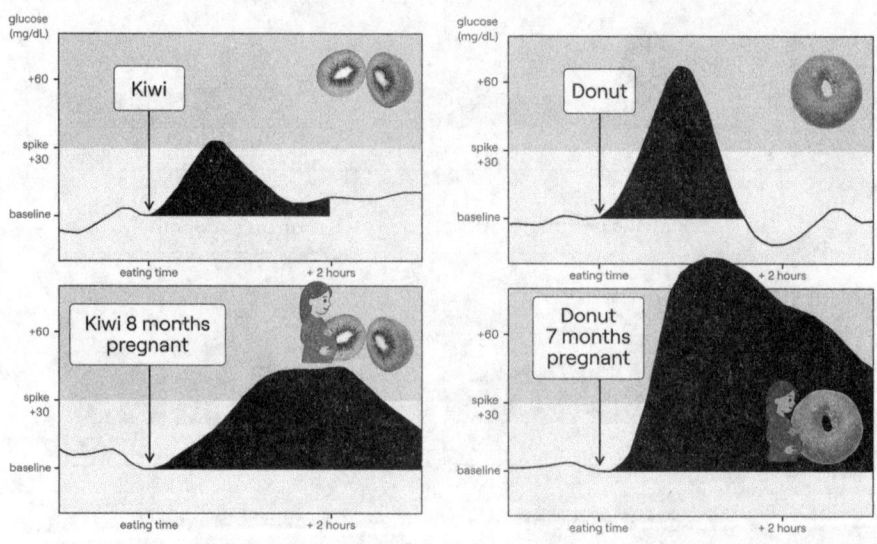

Insulin resistance adaptation will impact the glucose spike of anything that contains glucose: from a kiwi to a doughnut.

Now that you know how your glucose levels change during these nine months—lower fasting glucose levels, and longer and bigger glucose spikes—it's time to have a look at what's happening to your baby.

Glucose in the womb

Once your baby is connected to the placenta by the end of the first trimester, the more of any substance that is in your blood, the more your baby will have in his own. Whatever you eat, your baby "eats" too—glucose being no exception.

To prove this important fact, scientists have directly measured in-utero glucose levels in experiments, notably in one performed in Norway, at Oslo University Hospital.

During planned C-sections on 179 healthy mothers, researchers took a blood sample from each mother's arm just before delivery, and measured the glucose in it. (The moms had been fasting overnight, for at least eight hours, so these were their "baseline" or fasting glucose levels.)

Then, as soon as each baby was born, the researchers drew blood from the umbilical cord—which provides a direct, noninvasive way to measure the baby's glucose levels.

In each case, the baby's blood concentration aligned with the mom's: higher levels of glucose in the mom went hand-in-hand with higher levels of glucose in the baby, as the graph on the next page shows.

This means every cookie, every spike in your blood glucose, is echoed almost immediately in the glucose delivered to your baby. Remember, the placenta is not a barrier: it will just keep releasing glucose into your baby's blood, without regard for how much he *actually needs*. And considering what you have learned about the effects of high glucose levels, if you're thinking this might not be so great for your developing baby, you are correct. Keep reading.

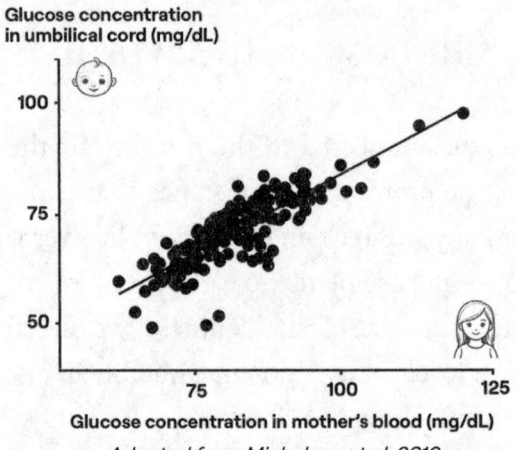

Adapted from Michelsen et al. 2019

Each black dot represents a mother-baby pair. The graph shows that the higher a mother's blood glucose level, the higher her baby's glucose level—demonstrating how glucose readily crosses the placenta.

Do we know how much glucose your baby requires during pregnancy? Less than you might think. In the third trimester, when he weighs about 6.5 pounds, scientists estimate that your fetus requires only about 35g of glucose per day. The placenta also needs a similar amount for its own energy. In total, that's around 70g of glucose—roughly the amount found in just **1½ cups (or 275g) of cooked rice**. That's it!

In the first trimester, there's no extra requirement: your baby is tiny and gets the minuscule amount of glucose he needs from uterine secretions. In the second trimester, the placenta is formed but your baby is still small, so the needs remain modest—likely less than the equivalent of a single cup of cooked rice per day.

This means that, **compared to the amount of glucose you ate prepregnancy, your need for glucose—or carbs—goes up by only the amount in less than 1½ cups of rice per day, and only**

in the third trimester. Meanwhile, your need for fructose (the sugar molecule that always travels with glucose in table sugar, fruit juice, and sweets) is **zero**: your baby doesn't need any.

So yes, in the third trimester it makes sense to add about 70g of starch to your day compared to the amount you were eating before—as long as your glucose levels are healthy and you don't need to restrict carbs to manage diabetes. 70g of starch is equivalent to: 1½ cups of rice as I mentioned, or two large potatoes, two cups of cooked quinoa, or two cups of cooked oatmeal. But there is absolutely no reason to eat more *sugars*. Of course, that's easier said than done, especially when pregnancy cravings hit. We'll look at cravings at the end of this chapter—how to understand them and how to handle them.

Which brings us to something that might have been on your mind since we first started talking about glucose levels during pregnancy: gestational diabetes, a clinical condition that can develop during pregnancy where you have glucose levels that are persistently too high.

The gestational diabetes test

When a doctor says the word "diabetes"—whether during pregnancy or not—it signals one thing: your glucose levels are high enough that action is needed to bring them down. As I said, while some glucose in the bloodstream is essential, too much brings side effects—not only to you but also to your unborn baby. This is well recognized in medicine, which is why gestational diabetes screening is now standard care.

To detect gestational diabetes, many care providers use the Oral Glucose Tolerance Test, or OGTT. In this test, you drink a liquid containing 50g, 75g, or 100g of glucose, and your blood is tested at different points: once before the drink (your fasting level), and again at set intervals afterward (generally 1 hour, 2 hours, and 3 hours after the drink).

The goal is to see how your body copes with glucose. Is your fasting level higher than it should be? Do your glucose levels spike too much after you take the drink—and stay high for too long? As I explained earlier, glucose spikes naturally become more pronounced during pregnancy. But in some cases, those spikes not only rise too high but linger, reaching a level where the side effects (such as inflammation in your body, which has a ripple effect of repercussions for your baby—more on this shortly) are urgent to address. If your fasting level is above 92mg/dL, or if your glucose levels are too high for too long after the test (above 180mg/dL two hours after drinking 75g of glucose, for example), you'll be diagnosed with gestational diabetes.

If you get the diagnosis, don't panic. Let's unpack it. For a long time it was believed that gestational diabetes happened randomly to some mothers during pregnancy. This could leave a mom feeling blindsided, wondering why her body had suddenly "failed" her for no apparent reason. But now we know better: in many cases, gestational diabetes is caused by preexisting high glucose levels and preexisting insulin resistance that simply become more pronounced and detected during pregnancy. How might this happen? One of the major factors is years of eating a diet rich in starches and sugars (one that repeatedly spikes glucose), which forces the body to call in insulin again and again to bring levels down. Over time, cells stop responding as well, resistance quietly builds, glucose quietly rises. So if you enter pregnancy already a little insulin resistant—and don't know it, because most of us are never tested (testing requires both fasting glucose and fasting insulin; see the Action Plan on page 71)—the added natural resistance of pregnancy can tip you over the edge into a diagnosis.

Recent studies confirm that gestational diabetes is often the continuation of a process that began before conception: one study from New Zealand showed that having a glucose level that is slightly high in the first trimester (when your glucose levels are similar to prepregnancy) predicts a later gestational diabetes diagnosis in 74 percent of cases. Similarly, a study on 700 women showed that a mom's frequency and height of glucose spikes at the end of the first trimester can accurately predict the condition.

Given that high blood sugar levels are not necessarily, as previously thought, entirely created during pregnancy, but may have been built by prepregnancy eating habits, they also don't always go away afterward: many women who get a gestational diabetes diagnosis continue to have prediabetes or type 2 diabetes after giving birth and after the pregnancy-induced changes have subsided. Note that for a smaller subset of moms, the diagnosis is not due to preexisting insulin resistance, but to a deficiency in insulin production.

Two takeaways here: first, if your prepregnancy diet contributed to high glucose levels and gestational diabetes without you knowing, this means that, by changing your habits, you can get your glucose down and manage the condition. The easiest path to this? Reducing the quantities of sugars and starches in your diet. Studies show that when women diagnosed with gestational diabetes reduce the amount of glucose they consume, their glucose spikes become lower, and their need for medication reduces.

And please know that if you do find yourself with a gestational-diabetes diagnosis, it's not your fault. Misleading marketing messages have led us astray: many foods labeled as "healthy" are actually terrible for our glucose levels and increase insulin resistance. In the Action Plan at the end of this chapter you'll find a list of foods that spike your glucose levels, so you'll be armed with information to make different choices. I'll also introduce my glucose "hacks"—that is, easy things you can do to reduce your spikes, so you can handle whatever comes your way.

Second, if a woman's glucose levels were checked in the first trimester of pregnancy, instead of in the third as is usually the case, she could find out ahead of time whether or not she is at risk for gestational diabetes, and make some simple dietary changes to do something about it. So ask your doctor to test your fasting glucose levels as early as you can during pregnancy to see where you stand (and if you are interested, also test your fasting insulin levels so you can estimate insulin resistance—in the Action Plan you'll find a recap on page 90 of blood tests you can run).

The important thing to know is that **a gestational diabetes diagnosis is not random, and it is not set in stone. You can improve your glucose levels and keep them in the healthy range, simply with what you eat**.

During my pregnancy, I chose to track my glucose very closely. I took monthly tests to check my fasting glucose levels, which were always below 92mg/dL, and I wore a continuous glucose monitor 24/7, which showed glucose levels never spiking above 140mg/dL. Combined with the fact that I was under 35, and my baby was measuring normally, my doctor and I agreed that the OGTT test was not necessary for me. (Not taking it is common in France, but in other countries the test is always mandatory.) But even so, I kept my glucose levels strictly in check—because they still mattered.

Here's why. The official diagnostic cutoffs aren't magic numbers. They are statistical markers, chosen based on population risk, rather than precise biological lines. **The impact of high glucose on both you and your baby doesn't begin suddenly at 92mg/dL. It rises gradually, step by step, as glucose levels climb.** So when you get your results, don't just look at whether you passed. Look at where you fall within the range. Being on the lower end is better for your baby than being on the higher end. Glucose may still impact your baby, even in the "normal" range.

From birth to adulthood

Your baby relies on the glucose you provide for energy. But as we just saw, he doesn't need that much of it. So, if you eat more glucose than your baby needs, the placenta will let it through, and your baby will receive an excess. And once excess glucose enters his bloodstream, he has to *manage it*. He registers all the same consequences as you do: stress in his mitochondria and inflammation in his little body. His tiny pancreas—less than an ounce at birth, about the weight of a raspberry—steps in to help, releasing insulin to lower his blood sugar. And just like in your own system, extra glucose gets stored in his liver, muscles, and fat cells. A little of this is normal and necessary, but repeated spikes push his system into overdrive.

The consequences of this are visible at birth: with each increase in a mother's glucose—even within the so-called "normal" range—a newborn's own glucose levels, insulin levels, and fat mass all rise too. Large global studies involving tens of thousands of women confirm this pattern: and it holds true **whether or not the mother had gestational diabetes.** Some babies are even born with such high glucose exposure that their blood already shows signs of insulin resistance. While a little baby fat is healthy, too much can signal that the baby has had to adapt to a stressful womb environment—protecting himself from excess glucose during pregnancy by storing it as fat.

That's the impact of glucose on babies in the womb. But what happens after they are born? It would be natural to assume that once a baby is out in the world, no longer exposed to his mother's glucose levels, his own glucose and fat stores would settle back to normal. But scientists have found *the opposite*. In large studies following tens of thousands of children, **those born to mothers with high glucose levels—or to mothers who ate large amounts of carbs during pregnancy—were much more likely to keep showing higher glucose levels and higher body weight later in life.** This is important, because it suggests that a diabetes diagnosis or obesity as an adult may trace back to the womb.

The evidence is significant: children born to moms with high glucose still had higher body weight at ages two, three, and four; a higher risk of obesity at five to seven; and higher odds even as teenagers. They were also up to eight times more likely to develop prediabetes or type 2 diabetes before the age of 22. This increase has been measured in many different countries: for example, in a study of 600 mother-child pairs in Denmark, 21 percent of children of moms with gestational diabetes got diagnosed with type 2 diabetes before 22 years old, compared to just 4 percent in the general population. This is a big deal: a teenager diagnosed with type 2 diabetes statistically loses 15 years of life compared to his peers without the condition.

And the links continue into adulthood: children born to moms with gestational diabetes have a higher body fat percentage as adults, and are twice as likely to become overweight in their lifetime, and are also at higher risk of developing type 2 diabetes as they age.

By the way, a normal birthweight does not necessarily indicate a healthy womb environment: even if your baby is born at a normal weight (the WHO considers a normal weight as over 5.5 pounds and generally under 9 pounds), if you had deregulated glucose levels during pregnancy, your baby is at 30 percent higher risk of developing obesity in the first ten years of life.

Researchers also looked at mothers who had multiple children—some born during a pregnancy complicated by diabetes, others during a pregnancy without it. They observed that the babies who were in the womb when their mom had diabetes were about four times more likely to develop type 2 diabetes as adults compared to their brothers or sisters born from nondiabetic pregnancies.

This finding is striking because the parent's DNA hadn't changed between pregnancies, and the children grew up with the same parents in the same household. The key difference was whether the pregnancy itself was marked by high blood sugar. Which, again, strongly suggests that the womb environment may play an important role in shaping long-term diabetes risk.

Still, it's important to remember that the long-term effects we've discussed so far are observational: they show strong associations, but not absolute proof. To truly test causation, we'd need an experiment where some pregnant women were assigned to eat a lot of carbs to drive their glucose levels up, and others very little, while everything else was kept the same. Then, the children would need to be followed for decades, to track who develops obesity or diabetes. A study like that would give us the answers—only it would also be, of course, unethical.

But history has given us something close. In the mid-20th century, a natural experiment unfolded in the UK that provided powerful clues about how a mother's carbohydrate intake—specifically how much *sugar* she ate while pregnant—shaped her child's health for life.

The sugar-rationing "experiment"

Between 1940 and 1953 in the UK, the population faced sugar rationing. This was because disrupted imports and the prioritization of war supplies during World War II had led to limited resources, and the government needed to ensure fair distribution and prevent hoarding.

People were given a daily allowance of 40g of table sugar per person. That's the white powder used to sweeten foods and in baking, which contains both glucose and fructose. The serving was equivalent to about eight sugar cubes.

People's consumption of fat, protein, fruit, vegetables, and starches did not change dramatically during this period. They were still getting glucose from starches (bread, rice, pasta, potatoes); it's just that their *sugar* was rationed, and as a result they were consuming significantly less fructose.

Everyone, including pregnant mothers, ate fewer cookies, cakes, pastries, chocolate, sweets, jam, and so on than they would have during peacetime. And this meant that for the nine months they were in the womb, babies did too.

Decades later, in 2024, researchers reached out to 60,000 adults born between 1951 and 1956 (just before sugar rationing ended, and just after), and asked them to complete a survey about their current health. The results were striking: **those who had developed in the wombs of sugar-rationed mothers had a 15 percent lower incidence of type 2 diabetes** compared to peers whose mothers ate nearly twice as much sugar after rationing was lifted.

On top of that, the babies who were conceived and then spent the first two years of their lives during the sugar-rationing period, meaning they weren't given as many desserts and sweets when they started to eat solid foods, turned out to have even better health: 35 percent less lifetime type 2 diabetes and 30 percent less lifetime obesity. **The longer someone had restricted sugar intake, both in the womb and as young children, the greater their protection against diabetes and obesity.**

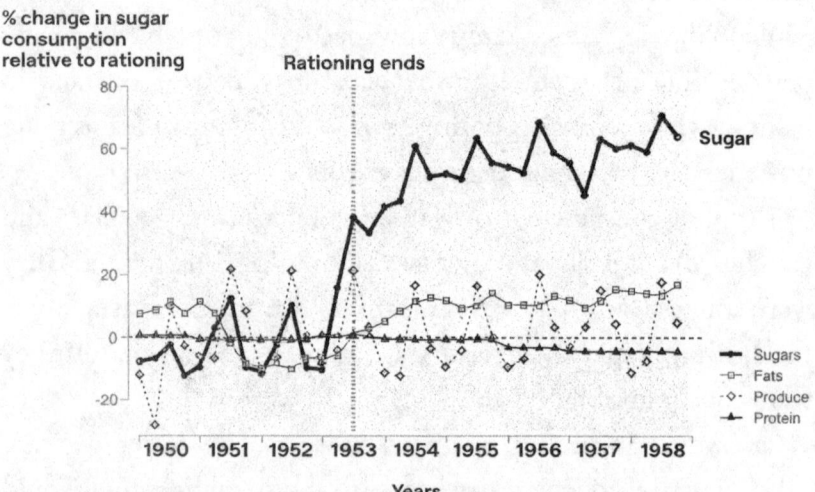

Adapted from Gracner et al. 2024

In September 1953, sugar rationing ended in the UK after 13 years. People quickly doubled their sugar consumption, and this had a detrimental lifelong health impact on the children conceived during that time.

These lifelong health benefits for babies were shown to come from just one change: their mothers having halved their sugar intake, from 80g to 40g per day. Less sugar meant lower glucose and fructose in both the mother's and the baby's blood, fewer spikes, less insulin, less inflammation—and children who grew up with a lower risk of disease.

This rationing data is considered unusually strong evidence

for a few reasons. First, sugar intake was controlled nationally, across an entire population, for more than a decade—a period during which pregnant women *had* to eat less of it, regardless of income, education, or lifestyle. Second, everything else in the population's diet stayed relatively stable. That makes it much easier to attribute differences in health outcomes to sugar itself, rather than to other confounders.

All the evidence so far tells a clear and consistent story: when pregnant mothers eat less sugar and keep their glucose levels in a healthy range, their babies are more likely to be born with healthier body composition, lower insulin levels, and a reduced lifetime risk of diabetes and obesity. Put simply, **eating less sugar during pregnancy protects your baby's long-term health.**

The World Health Organization (WHO) recommends limiting sugar to 50g per day, with 25g being even better (this includes the powdered sugar that comes in cakes, sweets, and fizzy drinks, and also the naturally present sugar in fruit *juice*, honey, and so on, but doesn't include the sugars naturally present in whole fruit). For perspective, that's actually less than was available during wartime rationing. But most pregnant women today eat far more. A US study of over 4,000 women found an average intake of 85g per day versus 77g when not pregnant—three times the ideal limit. Indeed, the numbers add up quickly: one cupcake or half a chocolate bar, or a glass of freshly squeezed orange juice contain 25g of sugar . . . *each*. **So, most mothers today consume sugar at levels that correlate with a higher risk of diabetes in their children.** Does this mean that if you eat cookies during pregnancy, your child will get diabetes as an adult? Absolutely not. But it does mean that eating one less cookie once in a while can ever so slightly nudge the odds.

Of course, sugar is also delicious, and in the tough early months of pregnancy in particular, it can bring real comfort (I know my chocolate croissants did). That's why, in the Action Plan at the end of this chapter, I'll show you how to enjoy it in ways that soften its impact on your glucose levels and on your baby's.

But for the moment, the big takeaway is that it's not just genes that shape our children's future. Clearly, our diet is also at play—passing on an increased or decreased risk of disease to our unborn baby. If you find this shocking, so did I. No one had told me this before. Suddenly, I looked at my chocolate chip cookie differently.

Now, I want you to understand exactly *how* this all happens at the cellular level. So grab your microscope—it's time to zoom in on the fantastic world of DNA, and talk about *epigenetics*.

The great DNA programming

When your baby was conceived, the genetic blueprint was set: half of the DNA came from you, half from the father. From then on, your child's DNA did not change.

But in the second half of the 20th century, researchers discovered something just as important. While DNA stays constant, small chemical molecules can attach to it and control how it works. These molecules act as switches, turning genes on or off. This process is called *epigenetics*.

And what controls these switches? Our environment. What you eat, how much you move, how well you sleep, the stress you experience, the chemicals you're exposed to—all of these influence the epigenetic programming that fine tunes how your DNA is used. For example, there is a gene called the LEP gene. This gene produces leptin—the hunger hormone that signals to your brain that you're full. The LEP gene can be epigenetically tuned up or down, depending on a variety of factors, which leads to more or less leptin produced—so the brain will get stronger or weaker satiety signals.

Today, epigenetics is reshaping medicine, from cutting-edge cancer therapies to gene-editing breakthroughs. And this field of science has also led to a revolutionary discovery of great interest to us that may start to explain the powerful associations we covered in the previous pages: a baby in the womb is *also* susceptible to these microscopic regulators. **The environment you expose your baby to during pregnancy** *dials his genes up or down*, **like a dimmer switch controlling a light.** Mind-blowing.

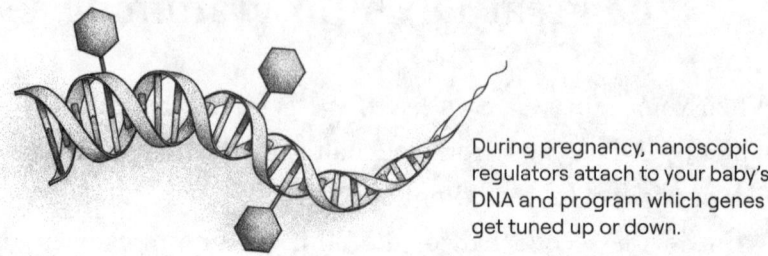

During pregnancy, nanoscopic regulators attach to your baby's DNA and program which genes get tuned up or down.

Researchers can measure this epigenetic programming in newborns by analyzing DNA from umbilical-cord blood at birth. A large study of 3,600 mother-baby pairs across the US and six European countries revealed something fascinating: babies born to mothers with gestational diabetes showed significant epigenetic changes on genes linked to diabetes risk. In other words, we have genes that contribute to our likelihood of getting diabetes, and these genes had epigenetic changes on them in children born to mothers with gestational diabetes. It means **the babies' DNA was programmed to be more likely to develop diabetes, starting inside the womb.** Even mildly elevated glucose levels within the so-called "healthy range" have been linked to epigenetic changes in newborns. This helps explain why, as we saw earlier, having elevated glucose levels during pregnancy led to a higher risk of diabetes in the babies. The high-glucose environment causes epigenetic changes, subtly steering the baby's body toward a lifetime of blood sugar problems.

Studies on rats, whose diets are precisely controlled by scientists, offer even clearer evidence. When moms without diabetes consumed a high-sugar diet during gestation, their babies had fat-storage genes activated, and fat-burning genes suppressed.

As adults, those offspring carried more body fat than peers born to mothers on a normal diet, even though *both groups ate the exact same food after birth.*

Remember the human studies we looked at earlier, where higher glucose or sugar intake in pregnancy was linked to children with more fat mass for decades? These rat studies help explain why: the babies were epigenetically programmed in the womb to store more fat and burn less. That "setting" stuck with them into adulthood.

All of this is compelling data about the epigenetic programming that occurs in the womb. And in case you still have any doubts that this is not just something a mother passes down to her children, regardless of her diet during pregnancy, hear this: siblings do not have identical epigenetic programming. Their epigenetic patterns differ based on their mother's health and glucose levels during each pregnancy. If during one pregnancy, for example, I ate only cookies, and in the other I ate no cookies, and much less sugar overall, my two children would have a different epigenetic makeup.

Breastfeeding also carries with it the potential to change your baby's epigenetics. Breast milk contains RNAs, which are one of the three types of microscopic regulators that attach to DNA and program it. Early research suggests that this might be one of the reasons why breastfeeding can have a long-term beneficial impact on a child's health. For example, a Dutch study looked at the epigenetic programming on the DNA of 120 children aged 17 months. It found that the less the child was breastfed, the more the gene that codes for leptin (the hormone I mentioned that makes us feel full after eating) was epigenetically silenced. This could potentially mean that these children ended up having lower leptin levels, hence more hunger signals after eating, and a greater tendency to overeat. In another study, children of mothers who had gestational diabetes during pregnancy showed two different outcomes: the babies who were breastfed had a 72 percent lower risk of obesity between two and four years old, compared to those who were exposed to gestational diabetes and were then formula-fed. One possible explanation is that the bioactive compounds in breast milk may have helped counteract, at least in part, the epigenetic changes triggered by gestational diabetes in the womb.

The conclusion is that, while the DNA your baby inherits is fixed, this doesn't mean your only option is to sit back and let nature do its thing. With every bite you take during the nine months of pregnancy, you have the chance to influence how those genes are expressed, and to actively set your baby up for success before he even arrives. **You are the *programmer* of your baby's DNA expression.** As I described earlier, scientists call this **"fetal programming."** It's a pretty astonishing idea to take on.

And please know that it is never too late to make a difference. Research shows that **when mothers with high glucose levels improve their diet and physical activity *during pregnancy*, they reduce their babies' epigenetic programming** toward these outcomes.

In addition, epigenetics are forever malleable: what your child will eat later in life is of tremendous importance. For example: perhaps my mom's pregnancy diet of breakfast cereal and mountains of sugar had something to do with why I landed on the cusp of prediabetes at 25. I will never know. But I was able to walk away from it: in my twenties I started using the glucose hacks you'll find at the end of this chapter. I went from borderline prediabetes to optimal glucose levels.

In short: **too much sugar, too often during pregnancy can nudge a baby's metabolism in ways that may matter later.** That said, I know firsthand how hard it is to cut back. Something about pregnancy itself seems to crank up those sugar cravings. Let's dig into why.

Can you program sugar addiction?

Why do we love to eat sugar? It comes down to *dopamine*, the "feel-good" molecule, which floods our brain when we eat sugar. It's the same molecule that gets released when we have sex, when we play a game, or when we get a notification on our phone.

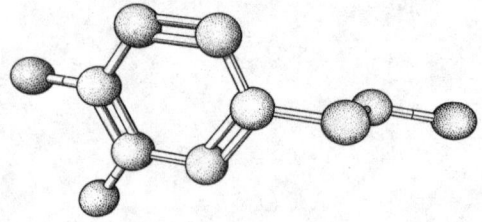
Dopamine

When you bite into a cookie and taste the sweetness of the sugar it contains, the part of your brain called the VTA (ventral tegmental area) immediately activates. Neurons in the VTA release tens of millions of these dopamine molecules in less time than it takes you to say the word "cookie." Dopamine then gets sent, in a hundredth of a second, through neural pathways to another part of the brain, the nucleus accumbens: the brain's pleasure center. This almost instantaneous two-step reaction is what makes you experience the pleasurable feeling associated with eating something sweet. Yum.

We like this feeling so much that we chase it. And that urge for more is what we call a craving. Scientists have long puzzled over why cravings seem to intensify during pregnancy: up to 90 percent of pregnant people report them—most often for ice cream, chocolate, and sweets. And as I mentioned earlier, surveys show that pregnant women eat more sugar during pregnancy than when they aren't pregnant.

THE COOKIE EQUATION

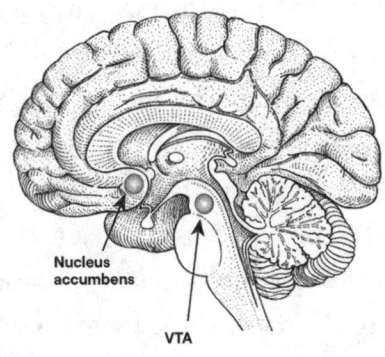

When we taste something sweet, the VTA in our brain releases dopamine within 0.1 seconds. Our nucleus accumbens then senses the dopamine within 0.01 seconds and triggers a feeling of pleasure.

Is this simply because we need more energy to sustain a growing baby, and that a craving for sugar ensures that we will seek out more food? Or is eating a lot of sugar during pregnancy perpetuated by a popular cultural belief that when pregnant "you're eating for two"/"you're going to gain weight anyway," so you should eat whatever you want? As it turns out, the answer may be more interesting. A 2022 study undertaken by scientists in Barcelona shed light on this mystery.

To understand what was going on, the researchers looked at the behavior of pregnant mice.

Like humans, the pregnant mice craved sugar: they preferred sweetened water over regular water. Brain scans showed that during pregnancy, their nucleus accumbens (the same part of the brain as the one we humans have, that senses dopamine) increased its number of dopamine receptors. This meant that, **while the mice were pregnant, the same bite of sugar triggered a *bigger feeling of pleasure*.**

This was an important discovery, and the scientists hypothesize that the same system is in place in humans. Regrettably, there aren't (yet) any studies looking at MRI scans of pregnant women and their dopamine receptors. But we do know this: during pregnancy, high hormone levels can make dopamine receptors in the brain more sensitive, so it's very possible that what was tested in mice applies to us. If this turns out to be true, it would mean that **eating a cookie during pregnancy makes us feel better than eating the same cookie when we are not pregnant.** Which could explain the cravings!

You may wonder: Isn't nature well made? Why would so many pregnant women have cravings for sugar if too much sugar might be harmful to their babies? It's possible that these pregnancy cravings exist to ensure the consumption of foods rich in glucose (such as fruit) whenever they are available, to make sure a mother has enough to sustain herself and her growing baby. A long time ago, when food was scarce, this could have been helpful. In our modern lifestyle, this adaptation has become detrimental because we have access to plenty of carbs, all the time—sugar and cookies are just far too abundant.

In the same mouse study on sugar cravings, scientists split pregnant mice into two groups: one with unlimited food (allowed to give in to their cravings) and one with controlled intake. The babies of the "all-you-can-eat" mothers showed subtle changes in their brain reward centers at birth and were later more likely to overeat when given unlimited food themselves. It seemed that craving sugar, and getting more pleasure from it, had been programmed in the babies.

Dozens of other animal studies echo this: offspring of mothers fed high-sugar or processed diets during pregnancy craved more sugar, sought more junk food as adults, and were more prone to addictions to alcohol, nicotine, and drugs like amphetamines and cocaine.

Scientists have found several possible reasons. First, glucose and fructose crossing the umbilical cord can cause **epigenetic changes in the baby's DNA,** turning on switches for stronger cravings and addiction-like behaviors. Second, excess calories in pregnancy may raise a baby's lifelong appetite, leading them to eat more than they need.

And finally, sugar's *taste* itself may play a role. By 12 weeks in utero, babies are already swallowing amniotic fluid, experiencing taste, and forming early flavor preferences. When you eat something sweet while pregnant, flavor molecules enter your bloodstream, cross into the amniotic fluid, and your baby swallows them. This could prime him to enjoy the taste of sweetness more, because what a baby tastes in the womb is thought to shape their predilections.

So when you eat many cookies, not only is your baby connected to you via the umbilical cord, receiving the glucose and fructose in them, which can over time influence his DNA, he is also tasting them and activating dopamine signals in his brain. In other words, if you are constantly eating sugar during pregnancy, you may be priming your baby to enjoy the taste of it more through two mechanisms—which might make it harder for you to ration the amount of sugar he wants as a toddler, and for him to ration the amount of sugar he wants as he grows up.

It's a double whammy: we crave more sugar when we are pregnant, and when we eat too much sugar this leads to bigger glucose spikes than usual, and both can affect our baby. It doesn't seem fair.

Still, it certainly helped explain to me why, during my first trimester of pregnancy, my diet consisted almost exclusively of chocolate pastries: I craved them and was too nauseous to eat anything else. But here's a piece of good news: **evidence suggests that it is during the third trimester that your baby's brain development is at its peak, and is most impacted by your diet.** In animal studies, if junk food in the rat mom is reduced during lactation (which is equivalent to the third trimester of pregnancy in humans, in terms of brain development), then the rat kids are less addicted to junk food (overall, they naturally eat 12.5 percent less junk food). So don't worry if you can't eat anything else but pastries early on: it's never too late in pregnancy to act on this information.

A note for after pregnancy: during breastfeeding, there is more leeway. By this point, as we've seen, you no longer share a bloodstream, and what your baby absorbs via your breast milk is not so directly linked to what you eat and drink. That said, if you eat a lot of sugar, studies show that breast milk, naturally sweet, can become even sweeter. That extra sweetness may further stimulate your baby's dopamine receptors and shape their taste preferences early on.

There is just one last thing we need to cover about how sugar affects your baby: the impact of inflammation.

Your baby's starfish brain patrol

As we saw earlier, eating a lot of sugar and having high glucose levels during pregnancy drives up inflammation in your own body and in your baby's, so different babies will be born with different levels of inflammation in their system.

The most common way to measure inflammation is with a simple blood test called the C-reactive protein (CRP) test. I know what comes next sounds confusing, but each lab has a different reference range: depending on where you get your blood drawn, a result below 5mg/L, 10mg/L, or 20mg/L may be considered "normal." Despite this, you should know that remaining on the lower end is better, as studies show that levels above 8mg/L start to be associated with complications such as preterm delivery (more on this in Chapter 4).

While he is in your womb, your baby's brain is growing at top speed—from zero neurons at conception to approximately 100 billion neurons at birth.

Amid this incredibly rich mesh of brain cells exist some vital companions: *microglia,* tiny immune cells that look like microscopic starfish. They are constantly surveilling your baby's brain for issues.

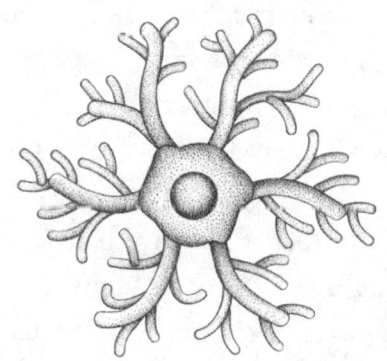

A microglia, the resident immune cell in your baby's brain constantly patrolling the environment, neutralizing pathogens and fixing damage.

If microglia detect a threat or a neuron that isn't developing properly, they shift into an **inflamed state**—rounded, blob-like, with retracted branches and a bulkier body. In this form, they engulf the threat and release inflammatory molecules into their surroundings. These molecules act like distress signals: they are picked up by nearby cells and spark a chain reaction of inflammation meant to fight off invaders and clear away damaged tissue.

A certain amount of inflammation is normal—even essential. Microglia use it to prune weak connections and eliminate faulty brain cells, sculpting your child's brain into a stronger, more efficient network. But glucose spikes can drive inflammation up too high and push microglia into a hyper-reactive state. When that happens, they may begin destroying neurons that should have been left intact. This misfiring can leave lasting imprints on brain development. Scientists believe that overactive microglia in a fetus's brain as a result of excess inflammation could be one of the reasons that **mothers with high glucose levels during pregnancy have children at higher risk of psychiatric disorders**. It's a connection rarely discussed, but the link is striking.

Let me walk you through some of the data. In Denmark, researchers tracked every single person born between 1978 and 2016: 2.4 million people in total. By age forty, 6.4 percent of them had been diagnosed with a psychiatric disorder. The scientists then asked a simple question: Were there any things about the mothers' pregnancies that stood out in these people? There were. Children born to mothers who had diabetes before pregnancy, or who developed gestational diabetes during pregnancy, were at a 15 percent higher risk of having *any* psychiatric disorder. Their risk of schizophrenia was 55 percent higher. Their risk of intellectual disability, 29 percent higher. Anxiety disorder, 22 percent higher. Developmental disorders such as autism and ADHD, 16 percent higher. Behavioral disorders, 17 percent higher. And to make sure the associations weren't explained away by other factors, the researchers controlled for parental history of mental illness, the child's sex, and the mother's age, weight, education, and whether she smoked during pregnancy. Even after all of that, the pattern remained: maternal diabetes during pregnancy was linked to higher risk in the child. Now, it's important to state that the overall prevalence of psychiatric disorders was low (as I said, it was 6.4 percent), and that most children born to mothers with diabetes did not go on to develop a psychiatric disorder. But the signal is there. And when studies this large line up with findings from others around the world, it should make us pause.

In another study, from Finland, researchers examined data from 1.2 million people born between 1987 and 2007. They measured inflammation in the mothers' biobanked blood during pregnancy and found that when C-reactive protein levels were in the highest quartile (above 5.8mg/L), there was a 43 percent increase in the likelihood of their child developing autism later on. This link between diabetes and autism in children was also confirmed in a 2025 review of 200 studies including 56 million mother-child pairs (yes, 56 million!). The researchers found that when mothers had diabetes during pregnancy, their children had a 25 percent higher risk of autism.

Inflammation of the brain is thought to be a leading factor in this connection, and epigenetics may also help explain why: babies born to mothers with gestational diabetes have autism-related genes epigenetically upregulated. Supporting this, animal studies and research on human brain cells in the lab also show that high sugar or inflammation in the womb can interfere with brain development, leading to ADHD- or autism-like behaviors.

Again, as so often when we are looking at human pregnancy studies, the results are associational, not proof of cause. And while the increases in risk are worth noting, they are relatively small in absolute terms. For example, a 25 percent increase in autism risk means prevalence rises from about 3 in 100 children (the US average) to about 4 in 100 among children of mothers with gestational diabetes. That doesn't mean gestational diabetes *causes* autism. It means that diabetes, and the inflammation that comes with it, is correlated with autism and could be one contributing factor among many. (Other pregnancy factors *correlated* with a similar increase in autism risk include vitamin D deficiency, and having low omega-3 levels—more on those in Chapter 4. Again, we don't have definitive proof for these, only observations suggesting possible links.)

And it's not all or nothing: the risk exists on a continuum. Research indicates that there is a correlation between the **severity** of maternal diabetes and the risk of neurodevelopmental disorders in children. For example, type 1 diabetes (which leads to the highest glucose levels) is associated with a higher risk of autism and ADHD compared to type 2 or gestational diabetes, as these types of diabetes lead to lower glucose levels than type 1. This suggests that any improvement in glucose levels would be associated with a lower risk of a condition in the child.

More research is needed on all of this, but what we do know is that inflammation during pregnancy—no matter the source—can affect fetal development. So it seems very strange to me that although a fever during pregnancy is treated as an urgent matter, as it signals acute inflammation or infection, which can be harmful to the baby if left unmanaged, as is preeclampsia (a condition marked by inflammation and high blood pressure), the chronic, low-level kind that stems from diet gets far less attention. **This is a great shame, because it is one aspect that we can actually do something about—simply by changing what we eat.**

To put the difference between acute and chronic inflammation into perspective, consider C-reactive protein levels, a marker of inflammation: while a high fever from an infection might raise CRP levels to 100mg/L, and a mild viral illness might raise it to 30mg/L, a single glucose spike after a meal might nudge CRP only from 1mg/L to 2mg/L (as measured by scientists in people with diabetes, the increase may be lower in people without the condition). This may seem small, but over time, a diet high in starches and sugars can shift someone's baseline CRP from 1mg/L to 5mg/L. And that low-level inflammation becomes the new normal. In fact, the study I mentioned earlier found that women with the highest levels of CRP (above 5mg/L—still far below infection levels) had a 43 percent increase in the likelihood of giving birth to a child later diagnosed with autism.

Again, that's not proof of causation, but it's a powerful signal that chronic, low-grade inflammation matters in some respect that scientists are still trying to uncover. And it deserves far more of our attention.

So let's recap what we know: During pregnancy, we often experience sugar cravings and reach for more cookies than usual. But this sugar now causes bigger glucose spikes than it normally would, leading to higher glucose levels in our baby's body, more inflammation in his brain, and more long-term consequences. The challenge is figuring out how to cut back without making life miserable—because the science we do have is clear: **this is not the moment to eat more sugar than we normally would.**

In the Action Plan following, we'll cover our first pregnancy building block: keeping our blood sugar levels healthy. I'll show you simple ways to manage your glucose levels and curb sugar cravings naturally, and I'll share strategies to solve what I call the "cookie equation": how—and when—to eat the cookie you want, with fewer consequences for your baby's health.

ACTION PLAN

1. Take a seat for sugar 101

Let's first cover what exactly *counts* as sugar—this substance that we are trying to reduce. While it might be obvious that doughnuts, sweets, fizzy drinks, cookies, and cakes contain sugar, there are other foods that we may think are good for us, when they are just as sugar-laden as the obvious foods, and lead to similar consequences on our glucose levels. (I've put a list of these foods on the next page.)

There is, though, one kind of sugar-containing food that we are always fine to have: whole, fresh fruit. Whole fruits contain fiber, which curbs the arrival of that fruit's sugar into our bloodstream. So if you are craving grapefruit and strawberries (I was!), go for it.

Here is a list of foods that you probably already know contain sugar:

→ Cakes
→ Chocolate
→ Cookies
→ Desserts
→ Fizzy drinks
→ Pastries

→ Sweets
→ White table sugar

Now here are the foods that you may think are good for you, but that actually contain just as much sugar as those on the previous list, and have the same impact on your body:

→ Agave syrup
→ Cereal
→ Cereal bars
→ Coconut sugar, brown sugar, or any other type or color of sugar
→ Dried fruit (dried mango, dried apricots, dried apples, raisins, and so on. And dried dates too—more on these and their impact on labor on page 228.)
→ Fruit compotes
→ Fruit jam
→ Fruit juice (even freshly squeezed at home, even with pulp)
→ Fruit smoothies (adding a little bit of whole fruit to a smoothie that also contains proteins, fats, and fiber is okay, but picking up a 100% fruit smoothie is just like picking up a can of fizzy drink)
→ Fruit-sweetened yogurts, such as a Greek yogurt "with strawberry pieces"
→ Honey
→ Low-fat fruit-sweetened anything
→ Maple syrup
→ Plant milks that have added sugar in their ingredients, or starches used as thickeners (such as rice starch—check the ingredient list on the back of the package)
→ Store-bought muesli or granola

→ And any product that boasts "made with 100% fruit sugar" or "100% fruit juice"

If this seems surprising, here is the deal: there is no such thing as "good" or "bad" sugar. Your body and your baby's body do not differentiate between the glucose and fructose molecules that came from table sugar and that are now in a cookie, and the glucose and fructose that came from an orange and are now in a glass of freshly squeezed orange juice. There is *no difference between the two*. Yes, the orange juice contains vitamins—but that doesn't do anything to slow how glucose is released into your bloodstream, or to curb the spike that follows, or mitigate the detrimental side effects.

If you think any of the foods in the list on the previous page are good for you, it's not your fault: decades of billion-dollar marketing campaigns have led you to believe it. This is the problem with the industrial food complex that is all around us today—messaging and health halos on packages are very misleading. But now you know better.

What matters when it comes to sugar is the **quantity of sugar,** and how it is delivered to your system: this is why a whole orange, complete with lots of fiber in it, is much better for you than a glass of orange *juice* (the sugar of three oranges, with no fiber to slow its absorption).

2. Understand what 25g of sugar looks like

Let's look at the WHO recommendation for daily sugar intake, which is 25g or below. The WHO is talking about the white table sugar that we add to things, along with the sugar naturally present in honey, fruit juice, dried fruit, fruit purée, and so on, that I have just mentioned. However, they do not count the sugar naturally present in whole fruit as being part of this recommendation—as I say, it's always okay to eat whole fruit. Below is a list of foods that contain about 25g of sugar. Eat any one of these foods, and you're at the upper limit of daily consumption. Just one glass of orange juice and you're done. Surprising, right?

→ 1 glass of freshly squeezed orange juice, with the pulp
→ 2 tablespoons of honey
→ 3 small chocolate-chip cookies
→ 1 cupcake
→ 8 squares of milk chocolate
→ 24 squares of dark chocolate (equivalent to a whole standard bar of 100g)
→ A small handful of dried mango

3. Choose starches over sugars

As I explained earlier, while your baby needs very little extra glucose in the first and second trimesters, he will need an extra 35g of glucose per day **in the third,** and your placenta about the same, which makes a total of 70g of glucose per day. But remember, it's much better to get this extra glucose from starches (bread, pasta, rice, potatoes)—or whole fruit—than from sugary foods (such as those in the previous two lists), which contain detrimental fructose too.

Here is a handy table of foods by type—sugar, starches, fiber, fat, and protein—showing which ones turn to glucose and which don't.

Mostly starch	Whole fruit	Mostly fiber	Mostly protein	Mostly fat
Contains glucose	*Contains glucose*	*Very little glucose.*	*Very little glucose*	*Very little glucose*
	Fine anytime	*Keeps you steady*		
Bagels	**Sugars**	Artichoke	Almonds	Avocado
Barley		Arugula	Brazil nuts	Butter
Bread (any)	*Contains glucose*	Asparagus	Cashews	Coconut milk
Breadsticks	*and fructose, no*	Broccoli	Cheese (any)	Ghee
Buckwheat	*benefit*	Brussels sprouts	Eggs	Olive oil (and
Cassava	Agave syrup	Cabbage	Fish (any)	any other oil)
Celeriac	Brownies	Carrots	Greek and plain	Pesto
Cereals	Breakfast cereal	Cauliflower	yogurts	
Chips	Cake	Collard greens	Ham	
Corn	Canned fruit	Eggplant	Hazelnuts	
Cornstarch	Caramel	Garlic	Macadamias	
Crackers	Cereal bars	Green beans	Meat and all	
Flour	Cookies	Kale	animal products	
Grains (any)	Corn syrup	Kale chips	Nuts (any)	
Granola	Crêpes	Kimchi	Nut butters	
Millet	Cupcakes	Lettuce	(unsweetened)	
Oat milk	Custard	Mushrooms	Nut milk	
Oatmeal	Doughnuts	Olive	(unsweetened)	
Oats	Dried fruit	Onions	Peanuts	
Pasta	Dulce de leche	Parsnips	Protein powders	
Pine nuts	Fizzy drinks	Peppers	Seafood	
Pita bread	(regular)	Pickles	Tofu and related	
Polenta	Frosting	Radishes	products	
Popcorn	Fruit juices (any,	Spinach		
Potatoes	even fresh and	Spring onions		
Pretzels	with pulp)	Swiss chard		
Quinoa	Golden syrup	Tomatoes		
Rice	Honey	Zucchini		
Rice cakes	Ice cream	. . . Any other		
Tortilla	Maple syrup	vegetable		
Turnips	Milks			
Sorghum	(sweetened)			
Squash	Milkshakes	**Fiber and protein**		
Sweet potatoes	Muffins	*Very little glucose. Keeps you steady*		
Wheat	Pastries			
	Pies	Black beans		
	Puddings	Chickpeas and other peas		
	Raisins	Kidney beans		
	Sweets	Lentils		
	Table sugar (any)	Soybeans		
	Toffee	. . . Any other type of beans		
	Waffles			
	Yogurts			
	(sweetened)			

4. Try fruit

A good way to reduce cravings for processed sugar? Eat whole fruit. If you give your taste buds whole fruit, you may very well satisfy that need for something sweet, and trigger your dopamine receptors without a big glucose spike. During my pregnancy I regularly added fruit as dessert—which helped me crave chocolate cookies less. Try a banana and peanut butter, an orange, a kiwi with yogurt, or whatever other fruit you feel like having.

→ In the recipes at the end of this book, you'll find some fruit-based desserts that often hit the spot for me.

5. Nip your cravings in the bud at breakfast

The best way to reduce your sugar cravings is to start your day with a *savory breakfast*. If you are having a breakfast that is made of carbs, such as oats with honey and a banana, toast with jam, or granola with orange juice, you will send your glucose levels skyrocketing first thing in the morning. It's the first dopamine release that will then leave you wanting more throughout the day.

And then, after that early spike, comes a drop. About two hours after your breakfast, as your glucose levels come crashing down, the part of your brain in charge of making you crave food will activate. You will want to find some sugar again—and this will create another glucose spike for you and for your baby, and then another dopamine release. If this is how your days start, it is near impossible to stand a chance against sugar cravings.

Because during pregnancy your body naturally develops increased insulin resistance, your spikes are higher, so your drops are steeper. This is another reason why your cravings may be increasing without you knowing it.

The antidote, as I say, is to have a **savory breakfast**. If you start your day with a breakfast built around foods that do not spike your glucose levels, you will keep your glucose levels steady for the rest of the day. Avoid the glucose roller coaster!

Refer to the table on page 75 to discover what these glucose-steady foods are.

Here's how to build a savory breakfast:

Make sure your breakfast contains protein. And no, this does not mean gobbling down ten raw eggs every morning. Protein can be found in Greek yogurt, tofu, meat, cold cuts, fish, cheese, cream cheese, protein powder, nuts, nut butter, seeds, and, yes, eggs (scrambled, fried, poached).

Also, add fat. Scramble your eggs in butter or olive oil, slice an avocado, or add five almonds, or chia seeds or flaxseeds to your Greek yogurt.

Extra points for veggies. I don't blame you if you aren't into veggies at breakfast. But if you can, try, as they will add beneficial fiber to the meal. I love mixing spinach into my scrambled eggs or tucking it underneath a sliced avocado on toast. Literally any vegetable, from spinach to mushrooms to tomatoes to zucchini to artichokes, sauerkraut, lentils, or lettuce will do.

Optional starch or whole fruit for flavor. This can be oats, toast, rice, or potatoes, or any whole fruit (the best option is berries).

Don't add anything else that is sweet. No honey, no dried fruit, no fruit juice.

When you start your day like this, you will not only feel fewer sugar cravings throughout the day, you will feel more energized and more satiated. Your savory breakfast should keep you full for four hours. If that's not the case, increase the protein.

Here are some no-prep savory breakfast ideas:

→ A bagel with cream cheese, topped with a few lettuce leaves or tomato and canned salmon
→ An apple with walnuts and slices of cheddar
→ Full-fat yogurt with sliced fruit, like a peach, a drizzle of tahini, and a sprinkle of salt
→ Greek yogurt swirled with 2 tablespoons of nut butter and a handful of berries
→ Half an avocado, dressed with lemon, olive oil, and salt, and 3 tablespoons of hummus with carrot sticks
→ Homemade granola that is nut-centric or cereal designed specifically with extra protein
→ Toast with almond butter
→ Canned tuna, a few pecans and olives, sliced radishes and cucumbers, a drizzle of olive oil
→ Toast with mashed avocado, goat cheese, and chile flakes
→ Tomato and mozzarella with a drizzle of olive oil
→ My go-to: leftovers from last night's dinner! (The fastest option of them all!)

Prep savory breakfast ideas:

→ Building Blocks Frittata (page 284)
→ Parmesan Fried Eggs (page 288)
→ A tortilla filled with black beans, chopped avocado, tomatoes, and onion
→ Full English breakfast (eggs, sausage, bacon, beans, tomatoes, mushrooms, toast)
→ Hard-boiled eggs, hot sauce, and sliced avocado
→ Pan-fried halloumi, sliced tomatoes, green salad
→ Poached eggs with a side of sautéed greens
→ Quinoa porridge topped with fried eggs
→ Sausage and grilled tomatoes
→ Scrambled eggs topped with crumbled goat cheese
→ Toast topped with fried eggs
→ Warm lentils topped with fried eggs

In the recipes at the end of this book, you'll find some of my favorite savory breakfast ideas.

✶ TOP TIP FOR MORNING SICKNESS ✶

If you feel nauseous first thing in the morning, try eating a small container of Greek yogurt while lying down in bed. Or a handful of almonds like I often did, or a piece of hard pasteurized cheese. I know all you want is carbs, and that's okay—just try to have a little bit of protein beforehand if you can; that will help with your nausea and mitigate the corresponding glucose spike.

Frequently Asked Questions

I'm finding it too hard to switch to a savory breakfast: What can I do?
Try making the switch in two steps: first, continue with your sweet breakfast, but have it *after* you eat some protein. For example, if you are used to porridge and honey, have some Greek yogurt or some scrambled eggs first. This is important because eating protein first slows the digestion of carbs that come right afterward, which will also keep you full—et voilà, smaller glucose spike. Then, over time, you can try to reduce the sugary part of your breakfast.

What about coffee, tea, and milks and glucose spikes?
We will cover drinks such as coffee and tea in Chapter 5. But in brief: the best milks to drink are regular dairy (whole—you don't need to eat skimmed or fat-free dairy, the natural fats are great for your glucose and will keep you feeling more full) and unsweetened nut milks (unsweetened almond, coconut, and so on). The milks that cause glucose spikes are oat milk (oat is starch) or any milks that contain added sugar (always check the list of ingredients).

What about sweeteners?
Stevia or monkfruit are better than table sugar. But avoid other sweeteners—the likes of aspartame or Acesulfame-K aren't great during pregnancy.

What if I skip breakfast?
No matter what time you eat your first meal of the day, the same concept holds: make sure you break your fast with

something savory. During pregnancy it's important to be fueling up consistently to provide your body and your baby with everything they need—so ideally, don't skip breakfast. If you don't have time, just grab a handful of nuts, some pre-hard-boiled eggs, or a dish of Greek yogurt from the fridge.

6. Solve the cookie equation: have your cookie... and a smaller spike too

When you eat a savory breakfast, you immediately reduce your chances of ending up on a glucose roller coaster (something most of us are on, and which is amplified by the hormonal changes during pregnancy).

However, it is perfectly normal to still want to eat sugar—and potentially even more so when you are pregnant, as we've seen—because your brain releases dopamine when you do. Sugar feels good!

The cookie equation offers you ways of having your cookie (or any other sweet food from the sugars list) to get the dopamine your brain is after, but with a lesser impact on your glucose, insulin, and inflammation levels.

Here's how to do it:

→ **Avoid sugar on an empty stomach, eat it as dessert after a meal instead.** Plus, try out my "Sweet things" recipes at the end of the book, as they are lower in sugar than traditional desserts, and might just hit the spot while keeping your glucose levels steadier.

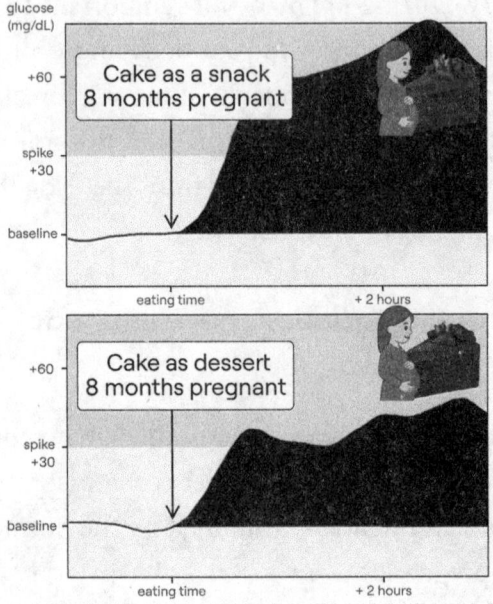

Sugar on an empty stomach is a recipe for a massive spike. Instead, have it as dessert and let the meal you just had slow down the absorption of the glucose in your bloodstream.

→ **If you are going to have a cookie or dessert after your meal, there is another thing you can do to lessen your glucose spike: think "veggies first."** Start your meals with an extra portion of veggies, or eat the veggies already present before the rest of your food. (When it's easy, and if you want to go the extra mile, you can also eat the protein second, and the carbs last. But again, do this only when it's easy. Otherwise, just add a veggie starter to your meal and eat your main like you normally would afterward.) The fiber in the veggies will create a protective mesh in your intestine, which slows the digestion of the carbs that come afterward, and reduces the glucose spike.

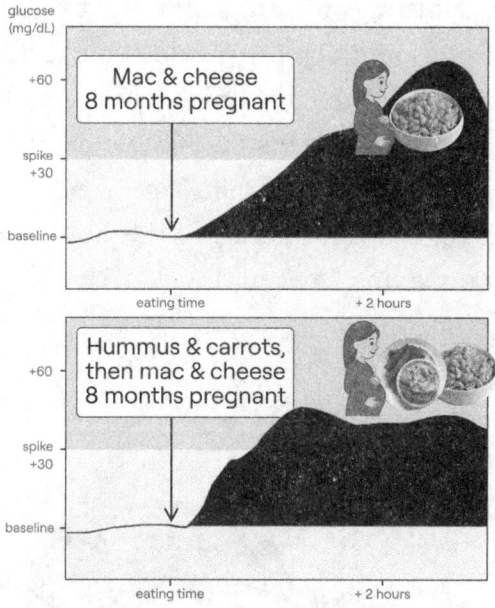

You can add some dressings or extra things to your veggies too—like the hummus here.

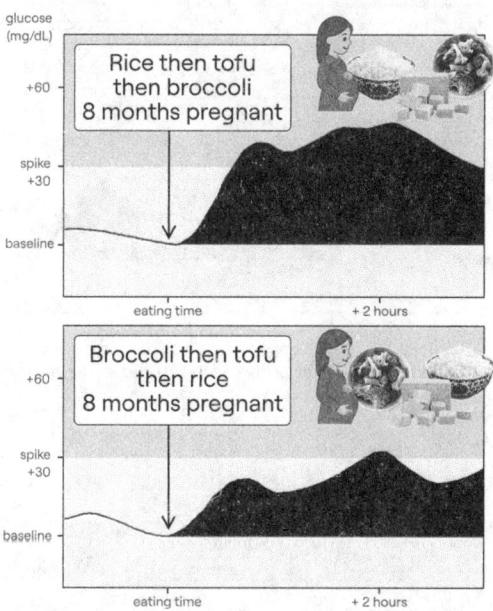

Same exact meal, different glucose spike—just by eating the veggies first and the carbs last.

→ **Add some "clothing" to your sugar.** That means don't eat any sweet food on its own. Add some protein, fat, or fiber to it (refer to the table on page 75 to find options for each category). So if it's the middle of the afternoon and you really want a doughnut, have it with some nuts, or a Greek yogurt. (At the end of this book you'll find recipes for satisfying "Sweet Things" that also apply this principle.)

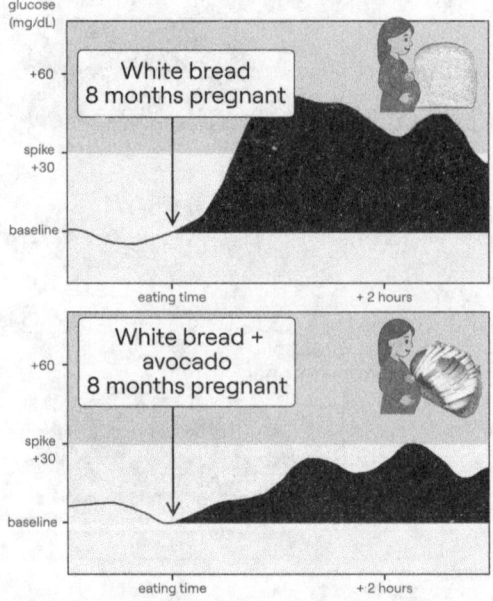

Adding clothing to your carbs isn't just better for your glucose—it often makes the meal tastier too!

→ **Move your body after eating sugar.** As you now know, all the cells in your body use glucose for energy, which means this is true for the cells in your muscles. We can use this to our advantage to reduce the spike that sugar creates: if within 90 minutes of eating something sweet, you use your muscles (go for a walk, clean your apartment, do some calf raises), some of the glucose you just ate will be absorbed by your muscle cells instead of staying in your and your baby's bloodstream.

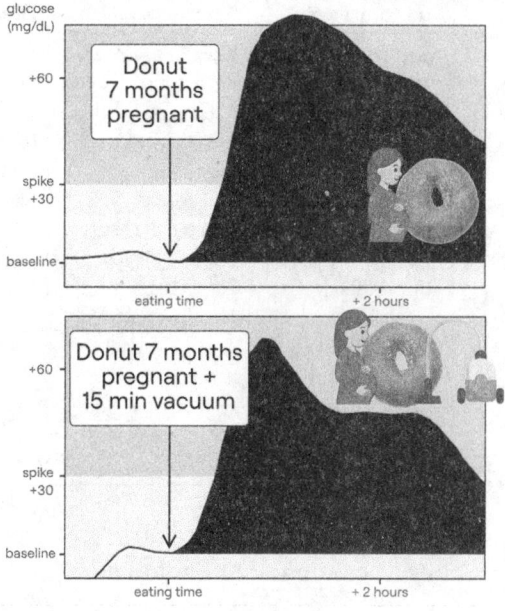

Any type of movement—walking or dancing or vacuuming—counts!

THE RECAP: TO AVOID A GLUCOSE ROLLER COASTER DURING PREGNANCY

1st trimester	2nd trimester	3rd trimester	Breastfeeding
Eat what you can if nausea hits. If you're not nauseous, keep your added sugar intake minimal and use the hacks to lower the spike.	Keep your added sugar intake as low as possible, and use the hacks to lower the spike. You need just a little bit of extra glucose: likely less than 1 cup (or 195g) of rice. Try to get it from starches instead of sugars.	Keep your added sugar intake as low as possible, and use the hacks to lower the spike. You need a bit of extra glucose: 70g per day, or 1½ cups (or 275g) of rice. Try to get it from starches instead of sugars.	Less important, but excess sugar intake can pass into breast milk. So keep doing the hacks if you can.

→ **Choose starches over sugars when you eat carbs.**

→ **Have a savory breakfast built around protein.**

→ If you can, focus on eggs as your protein source in the morning, which, as we shall learn in the next chapter, will increase your intake of an absolutely fabulous nutrient that is key to your baby's long-term health.

→ **Avoid sugary foods on an empty stomach,** eat them as dessert after a meal instead.

→ **Add some "clothing" to your sugar.**

→ **Move your body after eating sugar.**

✷ TOP TIPS ✷

✷ If you're nauseous in your first trimester and can't eat anything but carbs and sugars, don't feel guilty—do what you can.

✷ Build these tools as your pregnancy progresses, as your baby's sensitivity to your diet increases.

✷ Keep tons of whole fruits on hand at home. They are a good way to satisfy sugar cravings while keeping glucose spikes and inflammation low.

Frequently Asked Questions

Can I take vinegar while pregnant to lower the glucose spike? What about Anti-Spike Formula?
As long as the vinegar you use is pasteurized, it should be safe (choose white or red vinegar, though, because most apple cider vinegars aren't pasteurized—check the label). Adding a tablespoon of vinegar to a meal can lower its glucose spike. Anti-Spike Formula, my supplement that lowers glucose spikes by up to 40 percent, hasn't yet been tested on pregnant mothers so it's not recommended for the moment.

Is excessive weight gain in the baby during pregnancy explained only by sugar? How about overeating all foods?
Studies show that overeating unhealthy fats can also have bad consequences on the fetus, and can cause a baby to be

born with higher fat mass. High fat and high sugar usually go hand in hand in processed foods and desserts—so by focusing on reducing sugar consumption you should naturally reduce "unhealthy" fats, because they're found in these foods as well. It's also key to note that there are plenty of foods containing healthy fats that should be a part of your pregnancy diet, like olive oil, butter, animal fats, avocados, and nuts.

If I wear a continuous glucose monitor, what should be my objectives?
Speak with your doctor, but based on the cutoffs used for the standard gestational diabetes tests I used:

→ Fasting glucose, or glucose before eating/after having not eaten for two or more hours: below 92mg/dL
→ Two hours after eating: no more than 153mg/dL

Note that if you wear a continuous glucose monitor (CGM), the absolute value might be slightly inaccurate. These monitors don't measure glucose directly in your blood—they measure it in the fluid between your cells, which can differ a little from blood values. In fact, CGMs are usually about 10 percent off on average compared to a lab blood draw. Still, the patterns they show are reliable: they capture the rises and falls of your glucose, which is what matters most. Many pregnant women find that they don't need exact accuracy, but rather the overall patterns—where the spikes happen, how high they go, and how quickly they fall. For exact numbers, like your true fasting glucose or a precise post-meal reading, a blood draw or finger-prick device is still the gold standard.

What about eating dates, a dried fruit that is high in sugar, to help with labor?
There is interesting evidence that consuming six dates per day in late pregnancy does help with reducing the length of labor—but dates also create massive glucose spikes. Six dried dates contain 27g of sugar—the upper recommended limit of daily sugar intake. Personally, I did not consume dates, as the potential impact on labor did not outweigh the massive amounts of sugar and the glucose spike they create. More on this topic in our bonus chapter on labor and birth on page 228.

Blood tests and results

You can ask your doctor to run these tests during pregnancy, or depending on your country and healthcare system, you may be able to order them directly from a lab. Note that they are often not covered by insurance, so you may need to pay out of pocket.

Fasting glucose levels
Prepregnancy: glucose levels around 85mg/dL appear to be optimal. Higher than 100mg/dL is prediabetes.
During pregnancy: glucose levels around 79mg/dL appear to be optimal. Higher than 92mg/dL is gestational diabetes.

Fasting insulin levels
Under 5μU/mL prepregnancy is optimal. During pregnancy, the lower the better.

Measuring insulin resistance
To estimate how insulin resistant you are, researchers often use the HOMA-IR ratio (Homeostatic Model Assessment of Insulin Resistance). It's based on two simple blood tests: your fasting glucose and your fasting insulin.

The calculation is:

$$\text{HOMA-IR} = (\text{fasting glucose} \times \text{fasting insulin}) \div 405$$

The higher your HOMA-IR value, the more insulin resistant you are. A score around 1.0 usually means good insulin sensitivity, while values above 2.0 suggest some degree of insulin resistance (though exact cutoffs vary between labs and studies).

C-reactive protein
As low as possible prepregnancy. Note that this value can be impacted by many things other than just food: infections, pollution, chronic disease, and so on.

The gestational diabetes test
Depending on your country, or even your lab, you may be given a drink containing 50g, 75g, or 100g of glucose during your gestational-diabetes test. Your blood will usually be drawn before drinking it, then again one hour and two hours

later—although the timing can vary slightly depending on the protocol.

For example, here's what your results might look like for the most commonly used drink, containing 75g of glucose:

Fasting (before the drink): 87mg/dL
1 hour after drinking: 145mg/dL
2 hours after drinking: 110mg/dL

The official cutoffs for "passing" the test are as follows:

	Pre-drink, in the fasted state	1 hour after drink	2 hours after drink	3 hours after drink
50g glucose drink: often called the "screening" test or the "Glucose Challenge Test" (or "GCT").	Not measured, and no need to fast before the test	Must be below 130mg/dL or 140mg/dL	Not measured	Not measured
75g glucose drink: called the 75g Oral Glucose Tolerance Test or "OGTT" (this is the standard test used worldwide)	Must be below 92mg/dL	Must be below 180mg/dL	Must be below 153mg/dL	Not measured
	If ONE or more values exceed the cutoffs, gestational diabetes is diagnosed			
100g glucose drink: called the 100g Oral Glucose Tolerance Test or "OGTT"	Must be below 95mg/dL	Must be below 180mg/dL	Must be below 155mg/dL	Must be below 140mg/dL
	If TWO or more values exceed the cutoffs, gestational diabetes is diagnosed			

THE COOKIE EQUATION

In this example, of Fasting (before the drink): 87mg/dL, 1 hour after drinking: 145mg/dL, and 2 hours after drinking: 110mg/dL, the person has "passed." They don't have gestational diabetes as they remained below the cutoffs.

But the cutoff numbers (92mg/dL, 180mg/dL, and 153mg/dL in the case of the 75g of glucose test) are not magic lines. **They're statistical cutoffs, chosen based on population data to identify the point where the risk of complications starts to rise more sharply—not the point where risk begins.** A fasting (pre-drink) measurement in the 70s, for example, is more favorable than one in the high 80s. A one-hour result in the 120s or 130s is better than one in the 150s, and so on. The lower, steadier end of the range is where better outcomes begin—even before the clinical threshold is crossed. In fact, research shows that even mildly elevated glucose levels—still within the so-called normal range—can influence your baby's development: how they grow in the womb, how their metabolism adapts after birth, and even their long-term health. This is why I wrote this book: information helps to empower us, so we can put it in practice in a way that helps both our own body and our baby's development.

Cookie equation: solved. In the middle of a craving, implementing the hacks might not seem so easy to do, but rest assured—with time, these strategies will reduce how many cravings you experience, and will help buffer the consequences when you eat your delicious cookie. You might not use them every time of course, but getting in the habit can help.

Now that we've learned about the importance of managing glucose and fructose, let's turn to another substance. In this case, it seems your baby can't get enough of it.

CHAPTER 2

The six-egg problem

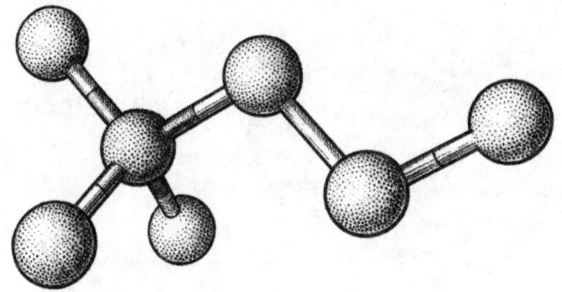

CHOLINE

THE SIX-EGG PROBLEM

It's time to meet one of the most underconsumed, underappreciated—and yet absolutely vital—nutrients in pregnancy: choline. You've probably never heard of it, but your baby's brain is counting on it.

As we have seen, to grow a baby in your uterus, you need to create one trillion new cells from scratch. Some will become liver cells, some retina cells, some brain cells, some muscle cells. Others will become bone cells, heart cells, blood cells . . . and so on.

Each of these cells is enclosed by a membrane, a thin layer that surrounds and protects it. This membrane is made of fatlike molecules called phospholipids, along with proteins, cholesterol, carbohydrates . . . and one other key component: choline. Without choline, the membrane cannot form.

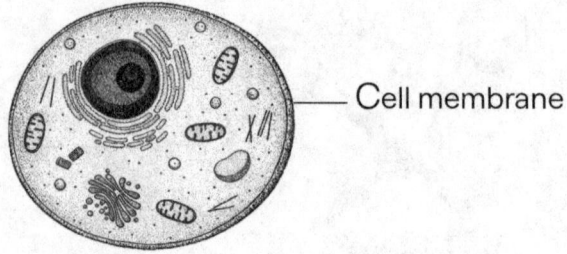

Choline helps form a cell's membrane.

To create a new cell, an existing cell must divide into two. And every time this happens, you need choline to make the new cell membrane. To be precise, you need *628 million* molecules of it per cell division. If you multiply that by the number of cells required to make a baby (one trillion), you get to a figure so large that I will spare you by not writing it out. (Well, if you really want to know, it's 628,000,000,000,000,000,000.) Suffice to say that during your fetus's development, the speed of cell division is higher than at any other point in life, **and as a result your choline needs during pregnancy increase significantly.** Just like your glucose passes through the placenta to your baby's bloodstream, choline follows the same route: your choline becomes your baby's choline.

But this crucial molecule isn't just important for your baby's new cell membranes. Enter: your baby's brain. Choline first helps form the neural tube (the precursor to the brain), it then helps create your baby's neurons, which will remain his neurons for life, as well as chemical messengers called neurotransmitters, which will enable his brain cells to communicate with each other. As the brain develops, brain cells need to migrate to their correct spot, multiply to the right number, and specialize into their final function. The supply of choline to your fetus's brain is vital for these steps to take place.

Choline helps develop the parts of the brain essential for **memory** (how well your child will remember things), **learning** (how quickly he will be able to store new information), and **attention** (how long he will sustain a task without getting distracted). Memory, learning, and attention: they're the foundations of your child's ability to navigate the world, build relationships, and thrive.

Finally, choline not only builds the brain, it can also protect it: in babies exposed to infections in utero, having more choline in the mother's blood may mitigate some of the negative consequences of such exposure on the baby's brain's development.

Indeed, during the nine months in your womb and the two years after birth (the so-called first 1,000 days), your child's brain growth is highly sensitive to the amount of choline available. That's why this molecule is a building block, and the focus of this chapter.

Beyond the building and the protecting, choline also helps with the epigenetic programming of your baby's DNA. As I explained in the previous chapter, your baby's genes are controlled by tiny molecular switches that turn the genes on or off. Choline is essential for the production of a type of switch called a *methyl group*. You must provide your baby with enough choline so that he can create the trillions of methyl groups that he needs for these switches to be created so that his genes work correctly. If you don't have enough choline, you can't keep up with that demand, and your baby's genetic programming may be affected. So choline has a double duty during pregnancy: it helps build each and every cell in your baby's body, and helps epigenetically program his DNA.

So how do we get hold of all this choline? Well, we can make some choline in our liver, but most of it comes from the foods we eat (more on that shortly).

Let's go back to the very beginning for a moment. Right after conception—once the small nutrient reserves stored in the egg are used up—your embryo depends on the secretions from glands in the lining of your uterus. These glands aren't created at the moment of conception; they were built and stocked in the months beforehand, shaped by your diet and nutrient status before pregnancy. (Which is why all of the information in this book can also be useful prepregnancy to help cultivate the best possible terrain for a potential baby to grow.) The uterine secretion contains molecules essential for early development, including choline.

Then, as we already know, around the three-month mark the placenta takes over as the main supplier of nutrients to your baby, sending them directly from your bloodstream through the umbilical cord. From this point on, what you eat starts to matter even more.

In fact, the placenta doesn't just pass nutrients along—it actively concentrates some of them for your baby. Levels of folate and vitamin C in your baby's blood, for example, run about one-and-a-half times higher than in yours. In the case of choline, it's even higher: studies find that your baby's blood can be up to *four times* more concentrated in this molecule than your own blood—yet another key discovery that shows just how important choline is to your growing child. (After birth, breast milk also concentrates choline. You'll find more details about breastfeeding in the Action Plan.)

Can you sort these blocks by color?

So we know that choline is essential for brain development in the womb. It plays a key role in forming the brain's structure and supporting its function. But researchers have gone beyond this well-known biological fact to look at real-world outcomes. In several studies, scientists have measured choline levels in pregnant women, then followed up by assessing various aspects of their pregnancies or of their children's development. By comparing maternal choline levels to the observed results, they've found correlations that are of great interest to us.

Being in the lower range of choline intake during pregnancy, for example, is associated with a 36 percent higher risk of neural tube defects, a brain malformation that usually ends in miscarriage. (Another more well-known cause of neural tube defects is folic-acid deficiency, which is why that supplement is often the main one recommended to pregnant women. See page 249 for more on supplements.) Studies have also found associations between low levels of choline during pregnancy and slightly slower brain development in the baby once he is born. For example, at 18 months of age, children of mothers with low choline levels were less adept at sorting blocks by color and shape and less capable of walking independently (common measures of coordination and problem-solving in toddlers) compared to children of mothers who had had higher choline levels. Another study found that children born to mothers with lower choline concentrations during pregnancy had slightly poorer memory at seven years of age, as measured with a memory game. Another study in women who developed an infection during pregnancy found that children born to mothers with lower choline levels had a harder time regulating their emotions at one year of age. Although these results might be influenced by other factors, they align with the understanding that choline plays a critical role in brain development in the womb.

Low choline levels can also have consequences for you, the mother. The placenta will draw as much choline as it can for your baby, even if that means leaving you short. When your own choline levels drop, this has real costs: your brain may not function as well as it could, and your cells can suffer damage. Without enough choline, cell membranes become more fragile, making it harder for tissues to repair and maintain themselves. Over time, this can contribute to liver dysfunction, muscle damage, and problems with memory or concentration. Insufficient maternal choline is also associated with a higher risk of preeclampsia and gestational diabetes.

It should be said at this point that the studies done on humans are all *observational*, meaning that scientists simply observed associations between low choline and these outcomes. They do not prove anything for certain or give us any precise numbers—such as, reducing maternal choline by 50 percent leads to 25 percent slower brain development. In order for researchers to be able to know for certain whether low choline *caused* these issues, they would need to do something unethical: they would need to deliberately reduce choline in the diet of one group of pregnant mothers and not in another, and measure the differences. These studies are not allowed, because we know that not enough choline is damaging.

With a little help from our rodent friends

While scientists cannot conduct randomized control studies on humans to determine the extent to which low maternal choline compromises a baby's development, they can experiment on animals, providing important insights. In 2016 at the University of North Carolina, researchers deliberately reduced choline to very low levels in the diets of gestating mice. They then observed the brains of the offspring under the microscope: they found fewer neurons being made in the brain overall, leading to smaller brain size, and brain development stopping earlier than it should. In another similar study, the low choline diet led to problems with retina development, the part of the eye that sends visual information to the brain. On the other hand, giving rodents plenty of choline during gestation was shown to have lifelong benefits in their offspring, such as maintaining good memory, improved attention, protecting the brain against damage associated with Alzheimer's disease, and reducing the severity of autism symptoms, epilepsy, and cognitive ageing.

As these studies show, fetuses *do not* automatically get as much choline as they need; and when there is too little choline, there could be consequences.

In other words, the fetus *does* depend on his mother's choline supply for his own development. If fetal choline levels were *always* optimal—completely independent of the mother's levels—we would *not* see these correlations between maternal choline levels and offspring outcomes in both animals and humans. The fact is that, depending on how much choline the mom has, the baby will receive more or less, and the impact of this is measurable. So much so that the American Academy of Pediatrics (AAP) stated that in humans, "Failure to provide [choline] during this critical period of brain development [the first 1,000 days] may result in lifelong deficits in brain function **despite subsequent nutrient repletion**." Basically, the AAP says that you cannot compensate later for a low choline level during this critical period, no matter how much choline your child eats as he grows older. I found it a bit scary when I read it. But here's the great news: getting enough choline isn't hard—eating a few eggs a day is the easiest solution (breakfast omelet, anyone?). And if you're not a fan of eggs, I've got plenty of tips in the Action Plan at the end of this chapter to help you get enough.

A shocking 10 percent

Recognizing the importance of choline for fetal development back in 1988, the US Institute of Medicine put a number on the recommended intake. It stated that pregnant women should get 450mg of choline per day, up from 425mg when not pregnant. During breastfeeding, they recommended 550mg per day, because you need 425mg for yourself, and 125mg passes through breast milk to support your baby's brain development (scientists can actually measure how much choline passes in breast milk). Across the Atlantic, Europe's public health recommendations date from 2016 and are similar (440mg, 400mg, and 520mg per day, respectively). These numbers constitute the minimum "adequate" recommended intake, and are agreed upon around the world—nothing controversial here.

We get choline from foods like animal liver, eggs, salmon, chicken, and to a lesser extent from plant foods such as broccoli and soybeans. As the studies show, choline is incredibly important, so you might assume that most pregnant women naturally consume enough of it. Well, this is where the numbers get shocking. Can you guess how many pregnant women consume the adequate amount? **Ten percent.** That is not a typo: *only 10 percent* of mothers-to-be eat the daily recommended 450mg of choline.

This statistic is from a large US national survey that assessed 25,000 people, and it is echoed around the world. In Germany, just 7 percent of pregnant women reach the recommendation. In Brazil, 1.4 percent. Canada does slightly better with 25 percent of women getting the adequate amount. The list goes on. Globally, the average intake is around 230–380mg daily. How could this be? One of the supposed reasons for this low intake is that choline is found in organ meats and high-fat animal foods—the best source of it being animal liver. And few people eat liver anymore.

> ## The lowdown on liver and pregnancy
>
> Just 25g of liver provides over 100mg of choline, along with other critical nutrients like vitamin B12, folate, iron, and vitamin A, all of which are especially important during pregnancy for your health and your baby's brain development. You may have been told to entirely avoid liver during pregnancy owing to its high vitamin A content and the risk of vitamin A toxicity (and problematic effects on the baby). But researchers have found that 80 percent of women in the US are actually deficient in vitamin A and not meeting the recommended intake per day. Additionally, the type of vitamin A found in food (retinol) is different from the synthetic versions linked to birth defects in old studies. According to current research, food-based vitamin A is safe in moderate amounts—and may even prevent birth defects linked to deficiency, such as problems with the baby's heart, lungs, and diaphragm. Based on animal studies and a few observational studies in humans, the maximum recommended safe dose of vitamin A is around 3,000mcg RAE per day ("RAE" is the unit used to express vitamin A activity). This is equivalent to eating about 85–115g of liver every single day. Which is a lot! Most health authorities now recommend a minimum vitamin A intake for pregnant women that translates to roughly 85–170g of liver

> per week (equivalent to 500–1,500mcg RAE of vitamin A per day depending on the type of liver), which works out to 25g of liver per day—or 100mg of choline daily. But because it's still a debated topic (and some countries cap liver to 50g a week during pregnancy), please get the all-clear from your doctor before tucking in.

If, as the data suggests, **the vast majority of mothers-to-be aren't getting enough choline to fully support optimal brain development,** this is absolutely not their fault. The importance of choline in pregnancy is severely under-discussed. Will their children be okay? Most likely, yes. After all, most humans alive today probably didn't get optimal choline levels in the womb, and most of us turned out fine. But "fine" isn't the same as optimal.

After reading these studies, I obviously called my mom and blamed her for everything that was wrong with my brain. No, I'm kidding. I just wanted to find out whether she had eaten enough choline while pregnant with me in the 1990s. I wrote down what she said about her diet and quickly did the math: Special K, Diet Coke, orange juice, low-fat meals (it was the trend back then), and just a few eggs. Conclusion: not enough choline. And listen, I didn't turn out too badly. I don't have any known cognitive deficits, but I do struggle with mental health, and studies find that vulnerabilities to adult mental health issues can have roots in what happened during pregnancy. Would my mental health have been better as an adult if my mother had eaten more choline? Would I be able to process emotions more efficiently and get less overwhelmed by stress? Would I be smarter? Who knows. Many pregnant women used to smoke cigarettes, and most of the children turned out fine, but when we found out that wasn't good for the babies, it became much less commonplace. Same thing here—once we have the information, we can act on it.

So the first thing to do is to make sure we get this adequate amount of choline during pregnancy. While animal liver is probably not on the cards, the second-best source of choline is eggs: one egg contains around 125mg of choline, so four eggs per day get you to 500mg, just above the minimum recommended 450mg. An easy morning scramble (and I have more options at the end of this chapter, if you don't like eggs). But the title of this chapter is "the six-egg problem," not "the four-egg problem." So what's the deal?

From four to six eggs

Here's the deal: 450mg might not actually be the best amount. That's because this recommendation comes from studies done not on the amount of choline that could create the most optimal environment, but on the *minimum* amount of choline needed to avoid problems. In other words, the minimum standard of soil for a tree to grow. Surely, though, what we want is the best, most fertilized soil so that the growing tree can be as healthy and majestic as it can be? Excitingly, evidence for how to achieve this is just beginning to come through.

Starting in the early 2010s, scientists designed studies to answer this question of whether more would be better. While it's not possible to restrict choline in pregnant mothers for ethical reasons (see page 102), it's ethically fine to give mothers *more* choline, because anything up to 3.5g (3,500mg) of choline per day is recognized as safe by the US Institute of Medicine and other global health organizations. (And don't worry, that would be very difficult to achieve—you'd need to eat 28 eggs per day to reach 3.5g.)

The researchers gave groups of pregnant women various high amounts of choline, and looked for any differences in their children's memory, attention and behavior (all areas of the brain that the scientists know choline plays a role in developing) *months or years* later.

For example, in one study from Cornell University on women in their third trimester, one group was given 480mg of choline per day (slightly above the bare minimum), and the other 930mg per day—through both food and supplements. The mothers didn't know which group they were in nor how much choline they were getting. They then graciously brought their children in for an assessment at four, seven, ten, and thirteen months of age. While sitting on their mothers' laps, the babies were shown a screen on which images appeared every few seconds. The babies who had developed in the womb of the mothers with the most choline had about a 10 percent faster reaction time to the images. This might seem inconsequential—after all, who cares how quickly a baby looks at pictures? Well, this test is used as a standard measure of cognitive ability because the faster a baby reacts to the images, the higher their IQ tends to be as a child and later as an adult.

But that's not all. The scientists brought the children back in when they were seven years old for two more tests: one a memory game and the other a test that required the children to stay focused for 12 minutes on an exceedingly boring computer-screen task. These tests are also used as standard measures—if you do better on them, you are statistically less likely to develop ADHD and dyslexia later in life. The results were interesting: children from the 930mg-choline-per-day group were better at both. This suggested that having more choline in the womb could lead to slightly better brain function, higher intelligence, and a lower risk of disorders—measurable *seven years after birth*.

The scientific community observed several things from this study: First, choline levels in utero can create lasting effects in the brain. Second, that the "bare minimum" might not bring brains to their maximal potential. And third, that even small increases may produce cognitive benefits for offspring (among the 480mg-choline-per-day group, children whose moms started supplementing earlier in their pregnancy showed slightly faster reaction times). So it might never be too late in pregnancy to get more choline. If you're in your 39th week of pregnancy, or if you're now breastfeeding, there's still time to make omelets.

In another study, this time at the University of Colorado and conducted by researchers who specialized in mental health, one group of mothers was given 900mg of choline in supplement form per day, from the beginning of the second trimester all the way to delivery. In addition, the babies were given 15mg of choline per day for the first three months of life. The other mother-baby group received a placebo: something that looked like these supplements, but wasn't. At one and three months old, all the babies were put through a test while they were sleeping: as they listened to a recording of auditory "clicks," the electrical activity of their brain was measured with a helmet (this is harmless and doesn't hurt; it's called an EEG). What the researchers were looking for was how their brains reacted when they heard two small clicks in rapid succession. Normally, a brain will respond less strongly to the second click. If it doesn't, this can be indicative of potential behavioral problems and an increased risk of the development of ADHD and even schizophrenia later in life. In the choline group, at one month old, the babies were significantly more likely to respond less strongly to the second click—a good outcome. Interestingly, when the same test was repeated at three months, there was no longer a measurable difference between the babies whose mothers had taken extra choline and those whose mothers hadn't. This doesn't mean the early benefit disappeared. Instead, it suggests that the control group eventually "caught up." The key insight is that choline seemed to accelerate the maturation of this brain function in the very first weeks of life, giving those babies a developmental head start.

At three years old, the scientists followed up with the parents and asked them to answer dozens of questions about their children's behaviors, like: "How much does your child fear doing new things?," "Are they cruel to animals?," "Are they patient about waiting?," "How easily are they frustrated?" The reason the scientists used this questionnaire is that the results are proven to be linked to future mental-health challenges. The children who came from supplemented mothers and who had received choline in their first three months of life scored better than those who had not received any extra choline.

These studies were small (26 and 100 mothers, respectively) and other studies designed similarly found *no difference* between the two groups. Research is ongoing on the topic of ideal choline levels above the bare minimum. However, the results point to some coherence: they align with what we know about how the brain forms in the womb, and echo 25 years of studies in animals. So while it is obvious that getting at least the bare minimum should be a goal for everyone, more could be even better.

One thing that is important to mention here is that in the studies cited above, the mothers were consuming choline in supplement form. And what was measured was simply the amount they consumed—the researchers did not measure choline in the mothers' bloodstream. Trials show that, as with many other nutrients, choline is marginally less well absorbed from supplements than it is from foods, so we may deduce that while 900–930mg may be optimum, we can still expect to see an impact on children's cognition at levels a bit lower than that when choline comes from food. In the Action Plan of this chapter (see pages 113–124), I'll go into more detail about choline goals and what you should aim for—but for what it's worth, my average daily consumption during pregnancy and breastfeeding was around 700mg, from food.

Unfortunately, given that only around 10 percent of mothers are reaching the bare minimum amount of choline today—whether it is consumed in food or supplement form—it's likely that virtually none are getting the levels that could potentially provide additional benefits. This is a problem, and again, it's not the moms' fault: in a survey of 250 healthcare professionals in the USA (obstetricians, gynecologists, midwives), it was found that only 6 percent of them speak about choline to mothers-to-be.

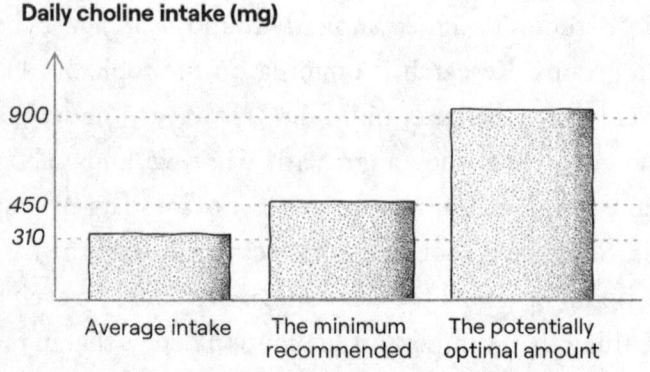

The potentially optimal choline amount is double the bare minimum recommendation, and almost triple the amount that most pregnant women consume.

A few times in this book I have mentioned the concept of "fetal programming": the idea that the environment in the womb can shape how a baby's genes are expressed and how their organs and brain develop. And the fact that if there is a limited supply of nutrients in utero, the fetus must adapt, which can impact his lifelong health. Diet is one of the key ways of programming your baby's future health, and given that eating more choline can have such important health benefits, it is a shame that more health professionals do not discuss it. Now is the time to get the word out.

ACTION PLAN

As you know, throughout this book we are putting together the most ideal pregnancy diet based on scientific evidence. So let's see how best to get this pregnancy building block: choline.

1. Learn how much choline you're consuming

A simple way to find out if you're getting enough choline during pregnancy is to take a real-life snapshot of your diet. Pick today (or yesterday) and, using the table on page 114, add up the choline in the foods you ate. Then record that figure at the bottom, and we will compare your total to the recommended amount.

Of course, your intake will vary from day to day, so this isn't a perfect measure. But it gives you a solid estimate. It's also one of the easiest ways to get familiar with which foods actually provide choline—because once you know where it comes from, it becomes much easier to include it regularly.

As you will see, there is much more choline in animal foods than in plant foods. This is because choline is concentrated in fats, which are abundant in fatty tissues like liver and egg yolks, whereas plants have less fat overall and rely more on fiber for structure. If you are not a big meat eater, or don't like eggs, don't worry! There are other ways to get your daily dose of choline. (Foods that aren't in this table aren't strong sources of choline in the diet.)

THE SIX-EGG PROBLEM

The food	Quantity of choline	How much of these foods do you eat on a typical day?
Animal foods		
Kidney (100g)	513mg	
Liver (100g)	290-420mg	
Chicken liver (100g)	290mg	
Egg, one	125mg	
Pork (100g, cooked)	100mg	
Salmon fillet (100g)	90mg	
Beef (100g, cooked)	80mg	
Oysters (100g; note that raw seafood is not recommended during pregnancy, but is okay during breastfeeding)	80mg	
Fish roe or caviar (1 tablespoon; note that raw seafood is not recommended during pregnancy, but is okay during breastfeeding)	79mg	
Fish or shellfish: cod, prawns, sardines and so on (100g)	75mg	
Chicken (100g, cooked)	75mg	
Whey protein powder (1 portion containing 20g of protein)	60mg	
Bacon (30g)	37mg	
Cow's milk (1 cup)	30mg	
Container of dairy yogurt	22mg	
Container of full-fat Greek yogurt (125g)	20mg	
Cream cheese, cottage cheese, or soured cream (100g)	20mg	
Mozzarella cheese (one ball, 125g)	17mg	
30g serving of cheese such as feta, cheddar, or pasteurized Parmesan (unpasteurized and soft cheeses aren't recommended during pregnancy but okay during breastfeeding)	5mg	

Plant foods		
Edamame (100g, cooked)	56mg	
Soy protein powder (1 portion containing 20g of protein)	54mg	
Soybeans (100g, cooked)	47.5mg	
Navy or lima beans (100g, cooked)	44mg	
Chickpeas (100g, cooked)	43mg	
Tempeh (100g, cooked	40mg (approx.)	
Broccoli (100g, raw)	40mg	
Brussels sprouts (100g)	40mg	
Cauliflower (100g)	40mg	
Collard greens (100g, cooked)	38mg	
Lentils (100g, cooked)	32mg	
Baked beans (100g, cooked)	31mg	
Peas (100g, cooked)	30mg	
Tofu (100g, cooked)	28mg	
Spinach (100g, raw)	22mg	
Pistachios (30g)	21mg	
Peanut butter (2 tablespoons)	20mg	
Peanuts, almonds or cashews (30g)	15mg	
½ avocado	10mg	
Zucchini (100g, cooked)	9mg	
A slice of toast or some crackers	8mg	
A serving of fruit: banana, blueberries, grapefruit, oranges, and so on	8mg	
Beetroots (100g, drained)	7.5mg	
Oats (100g, cooked)	7mg	
Flax seeds (1 tablespoon, milled)	7mg	
A serving of vegetables: carrots, cabbage, cucumber, peppers, tomatoes, and so on (100g, cooked)	6mg	
Pumpkin seeds (1 tablespoon)	5mg	
Tahini (1 tablespoon)	4mg	

Your total daily choline: ....

Your target goal could be anywhere between the bare daily minimum (450mg during pregnancy, 550mg during breastfeeding) and the potentially optimal amount (around 900mg), as suggested by the scientific studies based on supplements. I suggest you aim for at least 500mg during pregnancy.

2. Devise your choline strategy

If you like beef, chicken or calf's liver, they are by far and above the best source of choline. Personally, I can't stomach them. I tried—I promise. I even got some liver, cooked it, chopped it into tiny little pieces, froze them, and tried to take them as "pills." I was very motivated but this idea lasted a grand total of two days.

So my strategy was to max out the number of eggs that I ate per day. Eggs are a truly fantastic source of choline, on top of being a very healthy food and bringing many other nutrients. I can handle about four eggs in the morning (500mg of choline) as part of a savory breakfast (more on that soon), and sometimes an extra one (125mg) with my lunch or dinner. I often had a portion of meat, chicken, or fish during my other meals (150mg times two), and my go-to snack during pregnancy, as you'll learn in Chapter 3, contained a scoop of whey protein powder (another 60mg). With all that I regularly managed to get above 500mg, and most days I was closer to 700mg. (A note: during breastfeeding I had five scrambled eggs every morning, maybe more space in my stomach allowed me to easily eat one more egg in my breakfast.)

And if you're worried about cholesterol, don't be. More

on that in the Frequently Asked Questions at the end of this Action Plan.

Incidentally, while trying to conceive I took a prenatal vitamin that contained choline, and continued taking it during pregnancy and breastfeeding, but I didn't count this and used it more as an insurance policy. I tried to get all the choline I needed from whole foods (you'll find more on choline supplements below, and recapped in Supplements on page 249).

3. Make it last through breastfeeding

The importance of choline doesn't stop once your baby is born. During his first year of life, a baby has a "bare minimum" choline recommendation of 125mg per day from birth to the age of six months, and 150mg per day from seven to twelve months for adequate growth and development. And here again, a baby unfortunately won't just "get what he needs." The amount of choline in breast milk varies widely between mothers, with many having below this ideal amount. As you saw from earlier recommendations, breastfeeding is a time where your bare minimum intake of choline increases from 450mg to 550mg. Why is that? Because your baby's needs at this point are higher than ever, as his brain continues to grow exponentially after birth. And while we don't have the data on this, it's likely that even less than 10 percent of breastfeeding mums reach this threshold.

If your baby is formula fed, it's important to do your research: many baby formulas do not contain choline. So, check the ingredients on the package, and make sure that there is enough: 125mg until six months, and 150mg from seven to twelve months.

THE RECAP: TO GET ENOUGH CHOLINE DURING PREGNANCY AND BREASTFEEDING

1st trimester	2nd trimester	3rd trimester	Breastfeeding
450mg+ (depending on your level of nausea; if you can't eat choline-rich foods, it's okay)	450mg+ daily	450mg+ daily	550mg+ daily

→ If you can, **have a savory breakfast with four eggs.** I find this to be the easiest way to get choline in—first thing in the morning, you'll get 500mg, then you can forget about it. If you don't like eggs, try to add a portion of **meat or fish** to your breakfast. In the recipes at the end of this book, you'll find ways to keep eggs interesting, as well as some ideas for non-egg options.

→ **Make sure lunch and dinner contain a fish or meat source.** This is great for choline and for your protein requirements (more on that in the next chapter).

→ **If you are vegan or vegetarian,** consider a choline supplement to get your levels up. The most commonly used form is choline bitartrate. Some of the more cutting-edge prenatal supplements contain choline.

→ **During breastfeeding,** you can add fish roe and raw fish to your diet. While these aren't recommended while you are still pregnant, during breastfeeding they are safe to eat, and they contain a good amount of choline as you can see in the table on pages 114–115.

✶ TOP TIPS ✶

✶ Choline is in the egg yolk, not the egg white. So if you can't finish your eggs, just eat the yolk.

✶ If eating many eggs is difficult for you, consider scrambling them. By scrambling them, a lot of the water evaporates, so you have less food to eat overall compared to hard-boiled eggs, for example.

✶ Add an extra egg during lunch or dinner. Crack it into the pan as you're sautéing something, or soft-boil one to add to a dish of beans, pasta, or soup . . . eggs work especially well in these preparations.

✶ Your body cannot store choline that it's not using for very long, so you have to eat some every single day. You can't "stock up" on it. Having 20 eggs one day and none during the next few days doesn't work.

✶ If you can't imagine eating eggs in your first trimester because you are nauseous (like I was), don't worry. The first trimester is the least important with regard to your choline intake, as your baby is not yet connected to your blood circulation and needs only small amounts of nutrients to grow.

Keeping track of your progress: At the end of this book (pages 257–258), I have put together a daily checklist to help you keep track of your daily food goals. You can also download an extra copy and print it out at glucosegoddess.com/pages/9-months-daily-checklist or with this QR code.

Your daily checklist

Frequently Asked Questions

How on earth am I going to eat this many eggs?
I know, right? I hear you. I remember feeling overwhelmed by this too—like, am I supposed to live on scrambled eggs for nine months? Please know: it's okay if you don't eat enough choline. Nutrition in pregnancy isn't about hitting 100 percent of every target, every single day. What matters most is the overall pattern: if after reading this chapter you add in just one more choline-rich food per week (like one extra egg, or a few more bites of fish, or some beans) that's awesome. Just that is already helping you get more choline than you would have had otherwise. And remember: my mom ate only Special K, sugar, and Diet Coke. And I'm doing great (hey, I even wrote this book all by myself!). So no stress. Think of these recommendations as a compass pointing you in the right direction, not a rigid checklist you must follow perfectly. You're already taking an amazing step just by learning about this.

THE SIX-EGG PROBLEM

Aren't eggs full of cholesterol and bad for our heart?
When I told my midwife I ate about four eggs a day, she gave me a concerned look. This fear that eggs are bad for us—which is still unfortunately widespread—is based on very outdated information and trends that started in the 1970s. Today, scientists know that eating eggs is not bad for our heart—the cholesterol in them does not increase the cholesterol in our blood. In fact, **eating eggs is linked to a lower risk of heart disease**. And as of 2024, the US Food and Drug Administration (FDA) has officially re-categorized eggs into the healthy foods category. If you want a thorough recap of the latest science on eggs, check out my YouTube video on the topic. I've linked it here: glucosegoddess.com/pages/science-episode-eggs-and-cholesterol.

Egg science recap

Are eggs safe during pregnancy?
Yes, as long as they're cooked properly. The concern is salmonella, a bacterium that can sometimes contaminate raw eggs. While rare, infection can cause severe food poisoning, which is harder to handle during pregnancy and can, in rare cases, affect your baby. Runny yolks pose more risk, because the yolk may not get hot enough to kill salmonella. This is a conversation to have with your doctor, but here's what I did: I bought eggs from trusted sources, and when I soft-boiled them, I cooked them just long enough that the yolk was no longer runny, but gently set.

Cooking makes eggs safe, because salmonella can't survive high heat. That's why most health authorities recommend eating eggs only when both the yolk and white are firm. Another option is to use pasteurized eggs, anyway which have already been heat-treated to kill bacteria. You can usually find them in larger grocery stores (they're often labeled on the carton), and many restaurants use pasteurized eggs anyway for dishes like mayonnaise, sauces, or desserts. When eating out, it's worth asking if the eggs they use are pasteurized—most places will know and can tell you.

In short: eggs are a safe and powerful food in pregnancy—just make sure they're fully cooked, or use pasteurized eggs if you prefer them runny.

I don't eat eggs, what to do?
Prioritize meat and fish intake at every meal.

I am vegan/I don't eat any animal foods, what do I do?
Getting enough choline without eating any animal products is difficult. Make sure you're eating a lot of broccoli, peanuts, and soybeans. But even with those, you will not easily reach 450mg, and it will be near impossible to get the 700mg per day that I was reaching. You would need to eat 620g of dry soybeans (1.9kg of cooked soybeans, or about 2,700 calories of soybeans) per day to get 700mg of choline. So find a vegan source of choline in supplement form (for my recommended supplements, go to glucosegoddess.com/pages/supplements-pregnancy or scan the QR code below). If you are vegan because of ethical reasons, consider sourcing eggs from a free-range farm where birds are humanely raised. If you are vegan

because of health reasons, reconsider. A vegan diet, as you will continue learning in this book, is far from ideal for getting your pregnancy building blocks.

My recommended supplements

Can I take a choline supplement instead?
Some prenatal supplements contain choline, but most contain far too little. You can therefore supplement with an extra choline supplement (for my recommended supplements, go to glucosegoddess.com/pages/supplements-pregnancy or scan the QR code above), but do bear in mind that, as studies show, the absorption from supplements is not quite as good as from real foods. See supplements as an insurance policy, not as your main source of nutrition.

As I mentioned previously, in all the studies in humans I've cited, moms were given choline supplements. So it's very possible that they would have seen a similar positive effect by consuming less choline in food form, and therefore that we'd see an impact on children's cognition at levels lower than 900mg per day when obtained from food.

Is there such a thing as too much choline?
The recommended upper limit by the US Institute of Medicine is 3.5g per day (that is, 3,500mg per day). That would be about 28 eggs a day, which I don't think you'll get near to!

My baby is formula-fed, how do I make sure he gets enough choline? Make sure the formula contains choline (many don't). Check the amount of choline that is stated on the back of the package (usually under "vitamins") and choose a formula that has enough to allow your baby to get 125mg per day before six months, and 150mg per day between seven and twelve months, which is what he needs.

That's it for choline: now you know all about this fabulous, but underappreciated nutrient. It's time to move on to a much better known, if still relatively misunderstood, pregnancy building block for your baby's health: protein.

CHAPTER 3

The real body-building

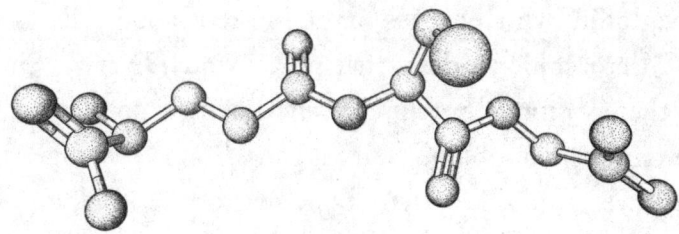

PROTEIN

Welcome to the protein section of this book. I know, I know, you're probably thinking: *I'm not looking to hit the gym and build muscle here, I'm busy enough as it is.* But protein is key to much more than just muscle. Excluding water, around 80 percent of your body is made up of protein. Or, I should say, protein*s* with an "s", because there are thousands of different types of them. Proteins play a crucial role in virtually all of the biological processes happening within you, from cell division to the creation of ATP, the energy molecules in your cells that we learned about in Chapter 1.

There are myriad substances in the human body that are in fact proteins: **collagen** that builds your skin and keeps it supple is a protein. **Insulin,** the hormone that stores glucose away, is a protein. **Antibodies** that protect you from viruses are proteins. **Hemoglobin,** which carries oxygen in red blood cells, is a protein. **Microscopic workers** that repair your DNA are proteins. And there's more. Proteins are the main components of your heart tissue, bones, blood, skin, organs, brain cells, digestive enzymes, eyes, immune system, bone marrow . . . and yes, of your impressive biceps too.

Your body is constantly making new proteins, and to do this it has to assemble a chain of 20 different types of tiny "pearls" called *amino acids* in various combinations, each with a name such as arginine, leucine, glycine, and more. These amino acids are so tiny that you could fit 600,000 of them side by side in the period at the end of this sentence.

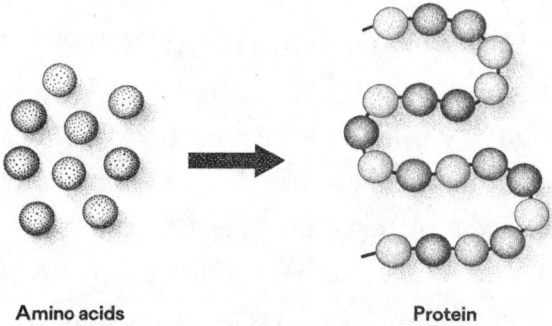

Your body assembles amino acids into chains that form proteins.

When your body needs a new protein—for example, some new **elastin**, the protein that enables your stomach skin to stretch during pregnancy—nanoscopic factories in your cells, called **ribosomes**, get to work. Ribosomes read the recipe for elastin from your DNA (well technically, from a copy of your DNA called mRNA—but we don't need to get into that here) and assemble the required amino acids in a chain to make it. Ribosomes work quickly, chaining about three to five amino acids per second, before sending the elastin away to perform its function: that is, to stretch your skin. Each cell in your body can make astronomical numbers of proteins per minute thanks to the millions of ribosomes it contains.

Now, in order to make all these proteins, your ribosomes need a steady supply of amino acids. Unlike glucose, however, your body cannot make all the amino acids that it needs from within. So you have to get them by eating protein-rich foods: eggs, dairy, fish, meat, pulses, lentils . . . The proteins in these get broken down into amino acids during digestion, to be used by your ribosomes. And, as I say, these amino acids are vital: without them, the machinery of life grinds to a halt. If you don't eat any protein, over time your ribosomes stop making all the molecules you need, and you eventually die.

Move over, Schwarzenegger

During pregnancy, your body goes on an extraordinary building spree. It creates new ribosomes that build your baby's placenta from scratch (the placenta contains 100 new grams of protein molecules), that enable your uterus to grow twenty times bigger (160 new grams of protein molecules by the third trimester), and increase your blood and fluid volume (200 new grams of protein molecules). But, your body is not the only one making new proteins around the clock—your baby's body is busy too.

In the very early days following conception, ribosomes in your baby's multiplying cells get to work: under instructions from his DNA, they build his bones, muscles, skin, joints, brain, blood, organs, immune system, and more. It is sometimes worth reminding yourself that inside your womb, you're building an entire human body. This is *real* body-building. And it's not happening in a gym for an hour a day—it's happening 24/7, fueled by what you eat.

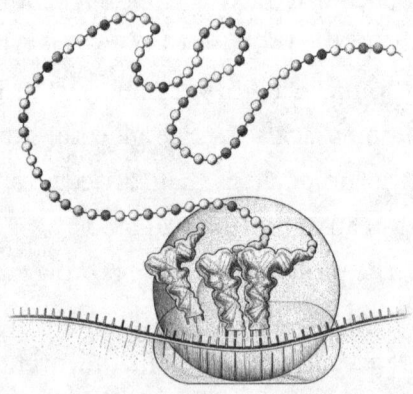

Proteins are made by ribosomes. This happens in you and in your baby. The protein you eat provides your baby's ribosomes with the amino acids he needs.

So when you're pregnant, you have two very hungry sets of ribosomes to power with the protein that you eat: both yours and your baby's need more and more amino acids as pregnancy progresses and growth accelerates. **Indeed, by the time he is born, excluding water, your baby will be made of about 50 percent protein.**

And here's the thing: to support this activity, **the amount of protein you eat during pregnancy must *increase*.** This may seem obvious but, as with the importance of choline and keeping your blood sugar levels steady, it is not something that we commonly discuss. So how much protein is enough? That's a question that scientists set out to answer.

A cutting-edge new technique

The first attempts to calculate precisely how much protein a pregnant mother needs to eat began in the 1940s. A technique called the Nitrogen Balance Technique (which compares how much protein you eat to how much you use) estimated that in the first trimester, a mother needs to eat 0.8g of protein per kilogram of bodyweight per day. This is the same estimate as for a non-pregnant adult, so 56g per day for a 155-pound woman like me would work out for example as: 3 eggs (21g), 1 salmon fillet (24g), and half a block of tofu (10g). For the second and third trimesters, the number was found to be 1.1g of protein per kilogram of bodyweight per day, which roughly corresponds to 20g of additional protein (an additional cup of Greek yogurt) to support growth of the baby, placental development, and the expansion of maternal tissue.

But, guess what? Science evolved, as science does.

While this technique laid the foundations of modern nutritional science, and was key during the 1940s and 1950s when researchers were trying to establish dietary protein recommendations, it's since been proven to severely underestimate our true needs. In the 1990s a new technique was born, called the Indicator Amino Acid Oxidation method (IAAO for short). This new method is so cool (nerd alert, I know). It works by tracking what happens to a special "indicator" amino acid in your body. If you're not eating enough protein, your body burns that indicator for energy. But as soon as you hit the sweet spot when your protein intake is high enough for all your needs, your body starts using that amino acid to build and repair tissues instead of burning it. It's a precise way to pinpoint exactly how much protein you need.

This cutting-edge technique found that adults actually need 1.0 to 1.2g of protein per kilogram of bodyweight per day to maintain their protein levels, not 0.8g/kg/day as previously thought. Similarly, it found that during pregnancy, a woman and her growing baby need much more protein than that advised by the Nitrogen Balance Technique:

→ First trimester: **1.22g/kg/day vs 0.8**
→ Second and third trimesters: **1.52g/kg/day vs 1.1**
→ Breastfeeding: **1.7–1.9g/kg/day vs 1.05**

Here, for example, is what these requirements mean for me, with the kinds of foods I usually like to eat:

→ First trimester: 1.22 × 70kg = 85g per day
    → 4 eggs (7g of protein per egg)
    + 1 chicken breast (40g per 140g of cooked breast)
    + a portion of cooked lentils (9g per 100g)
    + a small portion of full-fat Greek yogurt (8g of protein per 100g)
→ Second and third trimesters: 1.52 × 70kg = 106g per day
    → 4 eggs
    + 1 chicken breast
    + a portion of cooked lentils
    + a big portion of full-fat Greek yogurt (16g of protein per 200g)
    + 2 tablespoons of almond butter (7g of protein)
    + 2 tablespoons of grated Parmesan (6g of protein)

→ Breastfeeding: 1.9 × 70kg = 133g per day
  → 4 eggs
  + 1 chicken breast
  + a portion of cooked lentils
  + a big portion of full-fat Greek yogurt
  + 2 tablespoons of almond butter
  + 2 tablespoons of grated Parmesan
  + 1 salmon fillet (25g of protein per 120g portion)

(Head to page 156 in the Action Plan of this chapter to calculate your own needs, to convert pounds to kilos if you only know your weight in pounds, and to measure how much you are currently eating.)

So the amount of protein you need to eat during pregnancy is 50 percent more than was previously thought. You'd think pregnant moms might be informed about this, right? And yet, despite scientists calling for an update to the governmental recommendations based on this new technique, the general guidelines from health agencies have not been revised since the 1950s.

I don't know about you, but when I first calculated how much protein I was eating compared to my optimal amount, I was shocked by the gap. I consider myself quite a keen protein consumer, yet I was at only around 1g per kilogram of bodyweight per day. And the IAAO method leaves no doubt: **if we're eating less than its recommended amounts, we're in a state of protein restriction.** We may still be eating protein, just not enough to meet the needs of both ourselves and our baby.

And, clearly, protein restriction among pregnant women is common. When scientists compared IAAO targets to a US survey of 500 pregnant women, they found that in the first trimester, about 50 percent weren't reaching the optimal 1.22g/kg/day. From the second trimester onward—when protein demand surges, around 70 percent were falling short of the optimal 1.52g/kg/day. In other words, around 70 percent of pregnant women may not be consuming an optimal amount of protein from the second trimester onward.

If you're having twins or triplets, your needs will increase more, as you are building multiple bodies. Likewise, during breastfeeding, you'll notice that the amount of protein you need is even higher than in the third trimester. This is because your baby keeps growing once he is born, and you keep providing the amino acids he needs to grow through your breast milk. Your ribosomes create proteins to put into your breast milk, and your baby breaks these down during digestion, freeing the amino acids to feed his own ribosomes. (If your baby is formula-fed, formula contains the protein he needs, so after you give birth, your protein intake can go back to prepregnancy levels.)

I'll show you how to work out if you're meeting your own body's protein requirements later in the chapter, but first, we must look at what happens if those needs aren't met.

Doctor Barker

I have a confession to make. We're well into this book, and I still haven't properly introduced you to one of the most important figures in the field of pregnancy nutrition: Dr. David J. Barker, born in London in 1938, professor of epidemiology at the University of Southampton, father of five, warm, witty, and fascinated by beetles as a child.

In the 1980s, Dr. Barker found himself mulling over UK health records. One dataset showed heart disease deaths of adult men in the 1960s and 1970s. The other looked at the birth weights of those same adult men, dating back to the early 1900s. He noticed a striking pattern: baby boys born weighing less than 5.5 pounds had the highest rates of death from heart disease decades later. This was odd. According to medical wisdom at the time, heart disease was due to adult choices: too much rich food, not enough exercise. But the data in front of him told a different story.

So he pressed on with his research, and found more striking results: men in the UK who had been born with low birth weights (under 6 pounds) had the **highest risk of developing type 2 diabetes as adults** compared to those born heavier. Low birth weight was also linked to a higher susceptibility to high blood pressure, heart disease, and insulin resistance as an adult.

Being born small can signal that a baby has faced adversity in the womb—such as a mother having lacked adequate nourishment during pregnancy. For Barker, this data raised a radical idea: perhaps a suboptimal environment during fetal development could leave lasting marks, making these individuals more vulnerable to chronic disease later in life.

While fetal programming is familiar to you now because you've read the previous chapters of this book, at the time it was close to heresy. Barker was told his ideas were absurd, and he was rebuffed at every turn. This was not the kind of out-of-the-box suggestion the medical establishment welcomed. But he persisted, and finally, in 1989 *The Lancet*, one of the world's most respected scientific journals, published his findings.

Skeptical but intrigued, epidemiologists began sifting through birth records and adult health data from across the world, from India to South Carolina, China and Sweden . . . and everywhere they looked, lo and behold, the same pattern emerged. Babies who grew slowly in the womb, as reflected by low birth weight, were far more likely to face coronary heart disease, high blood pressure, type 2 diabetes, and stroke later in life.

Low birth weight can result from many factors: maternal smoking, illness, and poor nutrition among them, and can also stem from a baby being naturally small as a result of having small parents (in which case it's not an issue). In an attempt to isolate the role of diet, researchers now turned to history, searching for "natural experiments": moments when entire populations had endured sudden, severe changes in food supply, and where meticulous records had been kept. One such case stood out: the Dutch famine.

During World War II, the Nazis blocked food supplies to the Netherlands, and from November 1944 to May 1945 the country suffered a six-month famine. People lived on very few calories: 400 to 800 calories per day instead of the normal 2,000. Animal foods were extremely scarce. The intakes of proteins, fats, and carbohydrates plummeted.

THE REAL BODY-BUILDING

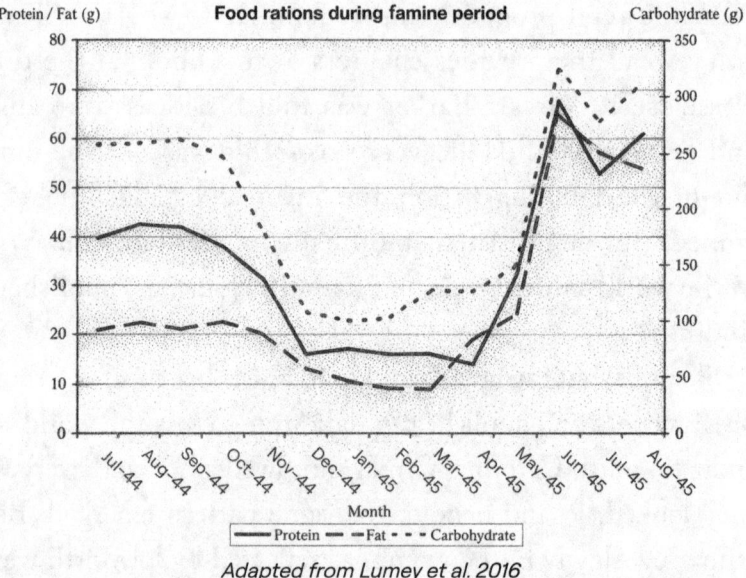

Adapted from Lumey et al. 2016

During the Dutch famine, food supply was abruptly reduced for six months, then went back to normal. The children who were in their mothers' womb during that period suffered lifelong consequences.

On average, babies whose mothers lived through famine during pregnancy were born 10.5 ounces smaller. Strikingly, long-term analyses revealed the same pattern Barker had described: these smaller babies experienced worse health outcomes for the rest of their lives, compared to those conceived just after the famine ended (and also compared to any siblings who weren't conceived during the famine). As adults, these smaller babies were more likely to have high fasting glucose levels or to have developed type 2 diabetes or obesity, and three times more likely to have developed cardiovascular disease. In addition, the female babies were five times more likely to develop breast cancer in their lifetime, and the males were twice more likely to have developed schizophrenia. Birth weights bounced back as soon as the famine abruptly ended, and the higher incidence of long-term chronic disease dropped.

The thrifty baby

How could a few months of poor nutrition in the womb leave such a lasting mark? Back in the UK, Barker and his colleagues had been developing a theory to explain their data. Their proposal was that when a fetus faces nutrient scarcity as he is growing in utero, he adapts for short-term survival—essentially "programming" his body to manage a resource-poor world. The trade-off is that, if that child then finds himself growing up in a world of abundance, those same adaptations can become liabilities. Barker and his team called their theory the **thrifty phenotype hypothesis**. ("Phenotype" is the scientific term for characteristic.)

According to this, **being born small is only the visible tip of the iceberg.** Beneath the surface, the baby has adapted to a limited supply of nutrients in the womb by making lasting changes to its metabolism and organ development. These adaptations may help survival in the short term, but they come at a cost: **the baby's body becomes "thrifty," meaning it is primed to store fat more easily, and it develops organs (like the pancreas, kidneys, and heart) that are more vulnerable to dysfunction later in life.**

Once Barker's theory gained traction, scientists set out to test it in the lab under controlled conditions. Success would signal that there was a biological basis for his observations—and that they were not merely coincidence.

Unable to do their trials on humans—which, again, would be considered unethical—the scientists embarked on a series of studies on animals, which enabled them to adjust one variable at a time, keeping everything else constant, to see how a mother's diet during pregnancy affected the baby. They aimed to discover exactly how the various different nutrients shaped development. The scientists studied many factors (such as calories and other micronutrients), but they noticed quite early that when one particular nutrient was restricted—**protein**—babies were born smaller. Unlike glucose (which your body can manufacture from other fuels) and fats (which are essential but your body can store for later use), protein has to be eaten daily—your body can't make it from scratch in the amounts you need. Furthermore, it is structural. It's the raw material for your muscles, your organs and even your hormones. As I described earlier, it powers the process of life day in, day out. You can't do without it.

The scientists' experiments followed a controlled protein-restriction model: take pregnant animals, feed one group all the protein they need during pregnancy, and give the other group only half. Keep calories equal by adding carbs or fat to make up the difference. Then watch what happens to their babies over their lifetime. Lo and behold, the results mirrored Barker's research: offspring born to the protein-restricted moms, were born small—whether rats, pigs, sheep, or mice—and grew up not only with lower muscle mass, but also with a higher risk of type 2 diabetes, high blood pressure, and obesity.

In most of these animal studies, as I said, when scientists lowered protein in the mothers' diets, they added extra carbohydrates or fat to compensate for the missing calories. Even so, the babies were born smaller, **showing that it was the lack of protein—not the lack of calories—that stunted growth.** This is very important: even with enough access to food, if the balance of nutrients is off, it can impact your baby.

In recent years, specific **mechanisms that explain this low-protein-worse-offspring-health effect** have been discovered through both animal and human research: when a mother is protein-restricted during pregnancy, her baby's pancreas (the organ that manages glucose levels through the release of insulin) develops with fewer cells than is optimal because of a lack of building blocks in the womb. This limits its capacity to fend off diabetes. Likewise, babies born with low birth weight are more likely to have incomplete kidney development, with fewer filtering units (nephrons), a deficit that can predispose them to high blood pressure later in life. In studies in baboons, where moms were fed 70 percent of the protein they would normally get during pregnancy, scientists found epigenetic changes that primed the babies' bodies to store more fat and to run on a lower metabolic rate after birth, conserving calories. They also found that brain circuits that regulate appetite became tuned toward stronger hunger signals. In childhood, all these adaptations might not cause any trouble, but you can see how later in life, after decades of strain on the body, they could make an adult more vulnerable to disease than his peers.

There have also been a number of observational research trials that give us additional insights into the importance of protein—**particularly for the developing brain**. In these studies, researchers group mothers by how much protein they reported eating during pregnancy, and then compare their children's outcomes as toddlers.

In a Chinese study of 1,400 mother-baby pairs, researchers found that moms whose diets were highest in protein and other vital nutrients during pregnancy had children with better neurodevelopment at three years old. Another study from Japan on 77,000 mother-children pairs found that moms with low protein intake during pregnancy (less than 9 percent of calories, or fewer than about 45g of protein per day) had children with a higher incidence of developmental delays by three years old: children born to these moms were less able to catch a ball, form sentences, and follow instructions. The children had a higher risk of communication delays (increased from about 4 percent to 6 percent risk), fine-motor delays (from about 8 percent to 11 percent risk), and problem-solving delays (from about 7 percent to 10 percent risk) at three years old, when compared to the children of moms who got more than 13 percent of their energy from protein (more than 65g on average). Scientists believe these observations stem from two things: epigenetic changes in the babies' brains owing to protein restriction, and a simple lack of amino acids—which are the building blocks of brain tissue and neurotransmitters. (Incidentally, good nutrition and stimulation after birth can help children catch up if they haven't managed to get everything they need in the womb, but studies suggest it rarely erases the effects completely.)

Thanks to Barker, who got the ball rolling, and the hundreds of scientists across the world who have added to the evidence, we can now point to consistent data results across species. Today, it is well established that when a mom is protein restricted, growth in the womb is compromised.

And that's not all: a fascinating new body of research has shown that protein restriction during pregnancy not only impacts your baby, it has consequences for you too. Because get this: if the placenta can't find the amino acids your baby needs in the food you eat, it won't simply give up, it will start taking them . . . from **your own body**. It will quietly raid your reserves, breaking down your muscles and siphoning off protein from wherever it can to keep your baby growing.

Bye-bye muscles

When your body senses that there aren't enough amino acids coming from food to support you and your growing baby, a response circuit is triggered called the Amino Acid Response (AAR) pathway. You can think of this as your body's low-protein alert mode. With resources scarce, the AAR pathway switches your body into conservation-and-recycling mode. Two things happen: First, your ribosomes are told to slow down and cut back on the production of new proteins. Second, your body begins breaking down existing proteins—pulverizing old, damaged, or nonessential proteins, and even entire cells—to release their amino acids and recycle them for your baby's urgent needs.

And where is the first place that existing proteins and cells get broken down? Your muscles. Muscles serve as your body's big protein reservoir, and their cells are sacrificed to free up amino acids. These then enter your circulation and get sent on through the placenta, to your baby's bloodstream to feed his ribosomes and help him grow. Muscles act like a backup pantry of amino acids when dietary protein falls short.

Many women lose muscle strength during pregnancy. In one study, scientists measured **hip muscle strength in pregnant women and found that 30 percent of moms had lost strength in this area by the third trimester, and 65 percent of moms had lost strength in it by one month postpartum.** This loss of strength as pregnancy progresses strongly suggests that muscle mass is being sacrificed in service of the growing baby.

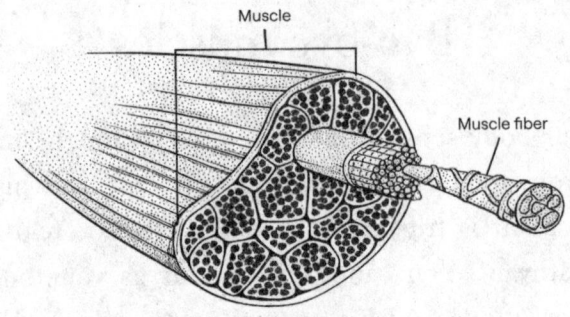

Muscles are often sacrificed during pregnancy if your baby needs amino acids to grow and there aren't enough coming from your diet.

While sacrificing your muscles is an amazingly helpful adaptation for your baby, it's not something to brush aside. Losing muscle during pregnancy can change your body composition, and it's not easy to rebuild unless you actively work at it. Research shows that postpartum, many women end up with higher fat mass and lower muscle mass than before, which sets the stage for a slower metabolism, long-term weakness, frailty, and loss of independence as we age. Muscle also acts as a storage space for glucose after you eat starches or sugars. If you are losing muscle as your pregnancy progresses, you are going to have less storage space—so the same cookie can trigger a bigger glucose spike, raising the risk of gestational diabetes and affecting your baby's glucose levels and epigenetic programming. This is why more muscle mass **is linked to a lower risk of gestational diabetes**, and also protects women who have had gestational diabetes from developing type 2 diabetes after they give birth. In short: we need our muscles.

Muscle loss during breastfeeding

When you are breastfeeding **your protein demands are even higher than during pregnancy**. That's because you need to eat a lot of it to produce the protein-rich breast milk that will feed your baby's ribosomes to continue his growth.

Breast milk is about 1 percent protein by volume (roughly 1–1.5g per 100ml). That may sound small, but babies drink a lot of milk, and the quality of that protein is incredibly high: it contains all the essential amino acids in the exact ratios your baby needs to build his body.

The proteins in breast milk come straight from you. Some, like casein and whey, are made in your mammary-gland cells using amino acids from your bloodstream. Others, like certain antibodies, are produced by your immune system and secreted into the milk. Every molecule of protein starts with amino acids you've eaten (or recycled from your own tissues), which are assembled by your ribosomes and packaged into milk for your baby.

In a study on rats, scientists found that during lactation moms lose 23 percent of their muscle mass. One quarter. **So if you've ever heard that breastfeeding makes you lose baby weight, please be aware that if you don't eat enough protein, it can also make you lose muscle.** You can imagine how one pregnancy can leave you weaker for the next pregnancy if you don't prevent muscle loss or compensate for it.

Animal studies back this up. In a typical experiment, one group of pregnant rats is fed an optimal amount of protein and the other group gets about 50 percent of that. All moms and babies are given the same healthy diet during lactation and adulthood—thereby isolating the impact of protein restriction to what took place in the womb.

In one of these studies from the University of Illinois, scientists found that **the rats on the low-protein diet had significantly lower muscle mass after giving birth**, and that the AAR pathway was twice as strongly activated in the muscles of those who were protein-restricted compared to the rats who ate enough protein. The researchers also saw that the **placentas** of the protein-restricted rats had the protein-recycling genes activated, suggesting that this organ was itself destroying some of its cells to give amino acids to the baby. As you can imagine this is not ideal, as a healthy placenta is important to a healthy pregnancy. An underperforming placenta means fewer nutrients reach the baby, adding yet another layer of growth restriction.

But here's the kicker: even with the mother breaking down her own muscles and the placenta sacrificing its own cells, it still wasn't enough to make up for the protein shortfall. At birth, the **babies of the protein-restricted rats were smaller than their peers, with smaller muscles and with signs of stunted growth.** We saw this in humans during the Dutch famine: when protein was restricted, babies were born smaller. The body tried to compensate, but it couldn't entirely.

And this story doesn't end at birth. Nine months of protein restriction leaves an imprint for life. The researchers found that the "muscle breakdown" genes were switched on in the pups' own DNA, and were still active when the pups reached adolescence (about 38 days old in rat terms). How does that happen? This is where epigenetics comes in. Remember, epigenetics is about tiny chemical tags—like methyl groups—that sit on top of DNA and act like switches, turning genes on or off. In these protein-restricted moms, an "on" switch was flipped during pregnancy in their babies' DNA, on the genes involved in breaking down muscle. These epigenetic marks didn't disappear when the pups were born. They stuck around, so when the pups grew, their cells kept following those same instructions: break down muscle for amino acids.

The AAR pathway response that the mothers experienced because of their low-protein diet had been imprinted onto their male babies. Why only in the male babies in this study and not the female? Scientists aren't sure, and we need more research to understand it. In another study in mice, scientists found that almost 1,000 genes in the muscles of babies (both male and female) born to moms eating a low-protein diet during pregnancy had undergone epigenetic changes potentially predisposing them to weaker or less efficient muscles later as adults. In the case of the Dutch famine babies, researchers found that a gene that's been linked to diabetes and obesity (called *IGF2*) was epigenetically changed to be more active—and this epigenetic change was detectable in the people that they tested 60 years later.

This is why scientists describe epigenetics as leaving a kind of cellular memory. The environment in the womb—whether rich or poor in nutrients—writes instructions on the baby's DNA. Those instructions can last well beyond pregnancy and may be difficult to switch off—even if protein and healthy food are plentiful after birth. Of course they *can* be modified by later experiences, but it means the choices you make now, big or small, have the power to give your baby a head start that will stay with them for life. That is the opportunity of these nine months.

Postcards to the womb

Let's imagine for a moment how a fetus prepares for life beyond the womb. Cocooned in there, he can't directly experience the outside world, so he relies on your body's signals—especially nutritional ones—to infer what kind of world awaits. And every meal you eat is, in effect, sending a daily postcard telling him about what it's like out there—how many resources, what he'll be able to work with, which building blocks are available. A diet rich in protein tells your baby: *"The world is abundant. You'll have all the amino acids you need to build strong organs and tissues."* A low-protein diet tells him instead: *"We don't have all the food that we need. Keep your muscles small, prioritize essential organs, store fat and prepare for scarcity."*

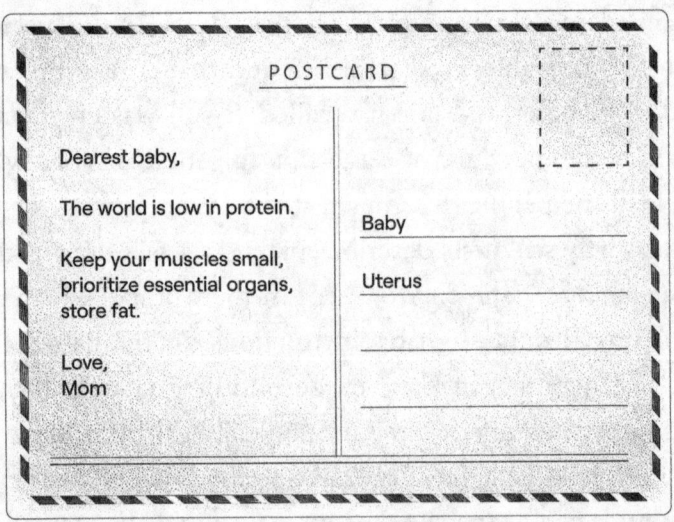

If you eat a low-protein diet, your body will send a signal to your baby to prepare for a world with low-protein availability, even if this is not at all reflective of the world into which he will be born.

These "postcards" influence how many cells his organs develop, how efficiently his metabolism runs, even how his brain's hunger circuits are wired. The wild part: **you don't even know that these postcards are being sent.**

The irony is that today, in many parts of the world, **protein isn't scarce at all.** If you aren't eating enough protein, it's not by choice or by lack of access, but rather a consequence of systemic lack of communication about this science. As we covered earlier, based on the IAAO results, 70 percent of moms are likely to be protein-restricted during pregnancy. We can be sure the vast majority of them aren't doing this on purpose. They just don't have the info, just like they don't have the info on the importance of choline or on keeping their glucose levels steady.

The stakes are high, the situation is preventable, and I find it all rather alarming that this science is not part of the standard of care in the medical system. Today, most moms are sending a message to their baby about protein that they don't even know is being sent. Their postcards don't reflect reality. And it's not their fault.

Likewise, you may remember from Chapter 1 how we discussed the problem of being overexposed in today's world to abundant, cheap calories—and how eating excess sugar and starch during pregnancy can set a baby up for lifelong metabolic issues. In this case, the message on the postcard we send to the womb will go something like this: *"The world is high in starches and sugars. You'll need to manage this big influx by storing more glucose as fat and increasing your insulin levels."*

Let's think about this for a moment: if you're under-proteined and over-sugared, which surveys indicate that many pregnant moms are, it's a double whammy of detrimental programming for your baby. Low-protein intake and high carbs actually tend to go hand in hand: when we eat little protein, we are hungrier, and we tend to reach for carbs to feel full. What do we need to do? Flip the script: optimal protein, normal levels of carbs. Avoiding the high-sugar low-protein pregnancy diet pitfall should be a priority for all of us. In the Action Plan, I'll share the steps I took to achieve it.

Now, a fair question might come to mind: Didn't we see in Chapter 1 that babies born large with a lot of fat mass—especially to mothers with gestational diabetes—are those who carry a higher lifetime risk of chronic conditions like obesity and type 2 diabetes? In Barker's data, the larger babies did not have an increased chronic disease risk—the smallest did. So which is it?

Both are true. The key is context, it's not size *itself* that matters, it's how that size occurred. If a baby is small or large *for genetic reasons*, and the mom ate enough protein, and the baby had all the amino acids he needed during development, risk doesn't increase with size. But if size reflects something else—like protein scarcity or excess glucose—then long-term vulnerability follows. **Up until the late 1980s, being born small was the leading focus for researchers looking at fetal programming. Since then, and with the rise in gestational diabetes worldwide** (in 2013, 14 percent of pregnancies were affected by gestational diabetes—in 2024, 15.6 percent, which is 18 million mothers per year, and the number keeps rising), **they know that fetal programming can occur across the birth-weight spectrum, and that babies born large because of glucose overload in their moms also carry risk.**

Incidentally, in his early work, Barker called babies born small "low birth weight babies." Today, the technical term for the extreme end of the birth-weight spectrum is a baby with

intrauterine growth restriction (IUGR) or fetal growth restriction (FGR): a baby who weighs 5.5 pounds or less at birth. The condition is defined as: "a complication of pregnancy where the fetus does not achieve its genetic growth potential." The risk of IUGR rises with lower protein intake. For example, in a study of 70,000 people, **vegetarian mothers** (who on average consume less protein than their omnivorous counterparts—more on that in the Action Plan later in this chapter) **were almost three times more likely to have a baby with growth restriction.** Today, it's well established (just as Barker originally uncovered) that, as adults, IUGR babies have increased risk of cardiovascular disease, metabolic syndrome, diabetes, respiratory diseases and impaired lung function, and chronic kidney disease.

Seventy percent of moms are likely not hitting their IAAO-based protein target. Does that mean that 70 percent of moms will have a low-birth-weight baby? No. The extreme diagnosis of IUGR is present in only about 10–15 percent of pregnancies worldwide. But it's not just about hitting a diagnostic cutoff. Even if your baby isn't labelled IUGR, low protein can still limit his growth. **In fact, research shows that with every decrease in birth weight—even within the range above 5.5 pounds—the risk of type 2 diabetes, cardiovascular disease, and high blood pressure increases.** For example, babies born at 6.5 pounds have a 12 percent higher risk for type 2 diabetes than those born at 7.5 pounds. What is clear, as shown in the animal studies we covered earlier, even moderate levels of maternal nutrient reduction are clearly sensed by fetuses and lead to changes in growth and metabolism. **Long-term increased incidence of disease is visible with even just moderate protein restriction (getting 30 percent less protein than you need).** If you are vegan, vegetarian, or relying on low-protein staples, your intake can quite easily drift close to that without you realizing it.

So, you're probably not going to have a baby with IUGR, but you could still be unintentionally programming him slightly toward scarcity if your protein intake falls short. Why not change that? In the Action Plan, we'll learn how to calculate your protein needs.

As a last point, I want to mention something important: several of my friends were told their baby was on the small side during ultrasounds. This can sound alarming, but being small does not automatically mean something is wrong. **How do you know if a baby is constitutionally small, as in naturally petite, simply following the blueprint of their genetics; or if a baby is experiencing growth restriction?**

Doctors look for specific red flags to tell the difference. On ultrasound, signs of true growth restriction include low amniotic fluid (a sign that the baby may not be getting enough nutrients or oxygen), abnormal blood flow in the umbilical cord or placenta, or a slowdown in growth over time, where the baby drops percentiles instead of following a steady curve. Maternal factors also matter: smoking during pregnancy, very low protein or calorie intake, or medical conditions such as high blood pressure can all increase the risk of restricted growth. When none of these warning signs is present, and the baby is growing consistently—even if measuring on the smaller end—the most likely explanation is a healthy, constitutionally small baby, simply reflecting the size of his parents.

I know this is a lot to take in. My goal isn't to overwhelm you, but to share the science so you feel empowered in your choices. And remember: even if your protein intake hasn't been ideal so far, it's not the end of the world. The increases in disease risk for babies with IUGR or lower birth weight are real but moderate, and healthy habits can offset much of that risk over time. Pregnancy and early life set the stage, but they don't dictate the ending. And the good news is, there are simple ways to boost your protein intake—I'll show you how in the Action Plan at the end of this chapter.

Now that you've seen the science, it's easy to see why we owe so much to Dr. Barker. Long before the evidence was overwhelming, he grasped what is now taken for granted: nutrition in pregnancy is one of the most powerful forces shaping lifelong health. Genes are not destiny—for example, barely 10 percent of type 2 diabetes risk lies in our DNA. The rest is dictated by our lifestyle and environment, including the prenatal one.

One of Barker's lines in particular has stayed with me: *"You live in two worlds—the world of your mother and the world into which you are born."* He passed away in 2013.

A friend with benefits

Eating sufficient protein has several positive domino effects. (And suddenly the Action Plans from Chapters 1 and 2 become far easier to achieve!)

First, protein doesn't increase your glucose levels. And when it's combined with starches or sugars, it lowers any glucose spike they'd cause. As I have explained, a protein-rich breakfast is a surefire way to avoid the glucose roller coaster for the rest of the day and reduce your cravings. In fact, there is a fascinating scientific theory called the **protein leverage hypothesis** that says that until you've given your body enough protein, it will keep you hungry: even if you eat bags and bags of cookies (nearly no protein in cookies), your brain will keep telling you to eat in the hope of eventually getting the protein it needs. Sound familiar? I've been there. Indeed, it is very common to be under-proteined and over-carbed: around the world, protein insufficiency is common, while true carbohydrate deficiency is extremely rare.

And this balance is important to get right in pregnancy, because the takeaway from all the available research is clear: **a low-protein, high-carb diet leads to worse outcomes for your baby than one with optimal protein and moderate carbs. And eating enough protein will naturally cause you to crave less sugar and starch, helping you and your baby on two vectors at once.**

The second advantage of a protein-rich diet during pregnancy is that **you are less likely to miss out on three other nutrients that are very important for you and your**

baby. The first is **choline**. Protein-rich foods are also rich in choline, a vital nutrient for your baby's brain development, as we saw in the previous chapter.

The second is **iron**. Iron is abundant in animal foods such as meat, poultry, and seafood, as well as in plant-based protein sources such as beans, lentils, and pulses. (Note that iron in plant-based sources is slightly harder for your body to absorb than iron in animal foods.) Your care team during pregnancy is likely to order a blood test to check your ferritin levels (which indicate your iron reserves—think of ferritin as your "iron savings account"). Higher in the normal range is better: mine was high before pregnancy (183mcg/L) and dropped to 38mcg/L in the third trimester, at which point I started supplementing with iron under the recommendation of my doctor.

Your baby needs iron to build his brain's structure. He will pull a lot from your body, which is why it's normal that your iron stores decrease as pregnancy progresses. But only up to a point: **a maternal ferritin concentration of less than 13.4mcg/L has been identified as an inflection point where your baby will not get enough, with potential long-term consequences on the development of his brain.** Iron deficiency in the womb has been shown to lead to epigenetic changes that persist through life, lower cognitive skills measurable at age seven to nine years old, and higher risk of heart disease as an adult. Some of these effects can be improved with iron supplementation during very early childhood, but certain cognitive deficits are harder to fully reverse. Low iron levels during pregnancy can have detrimental effects on your own health too—increased fatigue, shortness of breath, and potentially increasing the risk of preterm delivery and postpartum bleeding. Studies show that, on average, people who follow a vegan diet have lower ferritin levels, which is why it's even more important to be aware of this if you are vegan.

The third vital nutrient is **vitamin B12**, which is naturally found almost exclusively in protein-rich animal foods: fish, meat, dairy, and eggs. Today, with the increasing popularity of vegan and vegetarian diets, more and more mothers are being found to have low B12 levels. For example, a large study following 250 mother-child pairs found that by the third trimester, nearly one in two mothers were partially or fully deficient in B12. Unfortunately, this can have consequences for their baby's development.

At six weeks of age, infants of mothers with better B12 status were 2.4 times more likely to score in the top quartile for motor and language development. By age four, these differences persisted: children of mothers with sufficient B12 in the first trimester scored about 5–6 percent higher in working memory (a key skill for language, math, and problem-solving) compared to children of mothers deficient in B12.

Low maternal vitamin B12 intake during breastfeeding can also lead to low vitamin B12 content in breast milk, which can cause B12 deficiency in the baby. If left untreated, this can result in serious problems in brain and nerve development, such as developmental delays, movement difficulties, or vision problems (and if not recognized and treated quickly, can result in permanent neurological damage). Most prenatal supplements contain B12, but it's also important to get it through food, especially if you are on a vegan or vegetarian diet. If you don't eat animal foods,

THE REAL BODY-BUILDING

> look for fortified plant milks or fortified nutritional yeast. And do consider asking your doctor about having your B12 levels tested, which is straightforward.
>
> And one final advantage of eating enough protein: collagen and elastin, the two molecules that will help your belly skin stretch during pregnancy, are proteins. By eating enough protein you are helping your skin have all the amino acids it needs to stretch in the best possible way.

Now let's move on to our Action Plan and put everything together to make sure you are getting enough of our third pregnancy building block.

ACTION PLAN

1. Calculate how much protein you need to eat during pregnancy and breastfeeding

Science tends to favor the metric system, and that's what I follow, so the information below is in kilos. But it's very easy to convert pounds to kilos, and I'll talk you through it.

First, you need your prepregnancy weight in pounds. Then, convert it to kilos by dividing that number by 2.2. (Annoying, I know, but your phone calculator can come in handy here.) Now you have your prepregnancy weight in kilos. For example, if you weigh 154 pounds pre-pregnancy, like I did, divide 154 by 2.2 and you get 70 kilos.

→ Next, to get how many grams you need during the **first trimester**, multiply your weight in kilos by 1.22.

→ To get how many grams you need during the **second and third trimesters**, multiply by 1.52.

→ To get how many grams you need during **breastfeeding**, multiply by 1.9.

I've put a quick table of examples opposite in case you're reading this book on a desert island without access to a calculator (in which case, I'm jealous!). If your prepregnancy BMI is over 30, see my note below the table.

Weight range (kg)	1st trimester (1.22g/kg/day)	2nd and 3rd trimesters (1.52g/kg/day)	Breastfeeding (1.9g/kg/day)
40–49kg	49–60g/day	61–75g/day	76–93g/day
50–59kg	61–72g/day	76–90g/day	95–112g/day
60–69kg	73–84g/day	91–105g/day	114–131g/day
70–79kg	85–96g/day	106–120g/day	133–150g/day
80–89kg	98–109g/day	122–135g/day	152–169g/day
90–99kg	110–121g/day	137–150g/day	171–188g/day

→ **If your prepregnancy BMI is over 30** (the obese range), protein needs are calculated a little differently. (BMI, or Body Mass Index, is a simple measure: your weight in kilograms divided by your height in meters squared. For example: $70 \div 1.70^2 = 24.2$.) When BMI is over 30, using your full body weight can overestimate protein needs, because fat tissue requires less protein than muscle or organs. To adjust for this, you use an estimated lean body weight instead—about 75 percent of your actual prepregnancy weight. For instance, if your BMI is over 30 and you weigh 75kg, you'd use 100kg as your "lean" weight for calculating protein requirements.

2. Find out if you are protein-restricted

The best way to find out if you are meeting your pregnancy protein needs is very simple: take today as an example, and, using the table on page 158, add up what you ate and compare it to your protein requirement as we just calculated. Sure, it's not the most ideal way to measure this, as your diet varies day by day, but it will give a good indication. This is also a good way to get familiar with the foods that contain protein. (Note that foods that aren't in the table are not strong sources of protein in the diet.)

The food	Quantity of protein	How much of these foods do you eat on a typical day
Animal foods (all are complete sources, containing all amino acids)		
Chicken (100g, cooked)	30g	
Turkey (100g, cooked)	29g	
Beef liver or other organ meat (100g)	27g	
Beef (100g, cooked)	26g	
Prawns (100g)	24g	
Salmon fillet (100g)	22g	
Mozzarella cheese (one ball, 125g)	21g	
Can of tuna (100g)	20g	
Other fish or shellfish (100g)	20g	
Whey protein powder (1 portion containing 20g of protein)	20g	
Pork (100g)	18g	
Container of Skyr yogurt (125g)	15g	
Cottage cheese (100g)	11g	
Bacon (30g)	11g	
Container of full-fat Greek yogurt (125g)	10g	
Cow's milk (1 cup)	8g	
One egg	7g	
30g serving of cheese such as feta, cheddar, or pasteurized parmesan. (Unpasteurized and soft cheeses aren't recommended during pregnancy. During breastfeeding, no problem.)	7g	

Plant foods		
Pea, soy, or other plant-based protein powder (1 portion containing 20g of protein)	20g	
Tempeh (complete source, all amino acids; 100g, cooked)	20g	
Soybeans (complete source, all amino acids; 100g, cooked)	18g	
Edamame (100g, cooked)	11g	
Black beans (cooked, 100g)	9g	
Lentils (100g, cooked)	9g	
Chickpeas (100g, cooked)	8.5g	
Tofu (complete source; 100g, cooked)	8g	
Unsweetened nut butter (2 tablespoons)	8g	
Peanuts (30g)	7.5g	
Almonds, pistachios, or other nuts (30g)	7g	
Lima beans (cooked, 100g)	7g	
Peas (100g)	5g	
Quinoa (complete source; 100g, cooked)	4g	
A serving of vegetables: carrots, cabbage, zucchini, cucumber, peppers, tomatoes, spinach (100g, cooked)	4g	
Pumpkin seeds (1 tablespoon)	3g	
Hemp seeds (near complete source; 1 tablespoon)	3g	
Oats (100g, cooked)	2.5g	
Chia seeds (near complete source; 1 tablespoon)	2.5g	
Tahini (1 tablespoon)	2.5g	
½ avocado	2g	

Total average protein you eat per day: ....
Versus your optimal amount of protein: ....

> ## Why does it say "complete source" next to some plant foods?
>
> Most plant-based proteins are considered "incomplete" because they lack enough of one or more amino acids that our bodies cannot produce on their own. For example, grains are typically low in lysine, while many legumes are low in methionine.
>
> In contrast, nearly all animal-based proteins are complete, which makes it easier to get all essential amino acids from animal foods. Plant-based protein sources are "complete" when they naturally provide all nine essential amino acids in sufficient amounts—that is, amounts similar to animal proteins. Examples include: soy (tofu, tempeh, edamame), quinoa, buckwheat, amaranth, hemp seeds, chia seeds, and spirulina.

To clarify: **being protein-restricted does not mean that you aren't eating any protein.** It means you aren't eating *enough to reach your optimal amount*. Even if you eat eggs, fish, or a plant source of protein every day, you can still be protein-restricted if you don't eat *enough* of them. With an example diet of oats in the morning (15g of protein); a chicken breast, pasta, and vegetable salad for lunch (40g); some fruit and a cookie (0g); vegetable soup with some bread, cottage cheese, and pumpkin seeds (20g), you'll have around 75g of protein. If you weigh around 60kg, that's 1.25g of protein per kilo of bodyweight per day. Not bad, you might think, but this is below the optimal 1.52g/kg (which would take you to 91g of protein per day).

Remember: long-term increased incidence of disease is visible when a mom is eating just 70 percent of her optimal amount of protein. That's a moderate protein restriction (and when calculating your intake of protein vs your optimal intake, many of you will find that you are there). If you are vegan, vegetarian, or relying on low-protein staples, your intake can quite easily drift close to 70 percent of your optimal level or lower without you realizing it.

Maybe you won't hit the optimal protein intake every day. But that's okay. If you're eating with this goal in mind, and have a slightly more adequate intake than before reading this book, that's already fantastic. And remember—even if you are in your last month of pregnancy, it's never too late to make changes. Every day counts.

3. Make protein your main character

Instead of letting protein play a supporting role, give it the lead every time you eat. Anchor each meal or snack around it. During pregnancy, your glucose needs don't rise much—but your protein needs do, significantly. The best part? Protein-rich foods contain almost no glucose. So you can focus on getting enough without worry.

→ Make your breakfast savory (the recipes at the end of the book will show you how much protein is in them—I aim for about 30g per savory breakfast; they all keep your glucose steady, and I've also noted the breakfasts that help you get choline).

→ When you have a snack, build it on a source of protein, such as yogurt, tofu, a meaty leftover, and so on. I've included recipes for my favorite protein-rich snacks at the end of the book (especially my yogurt bowl, which I had almost every day; find it on page 304). They all keep your glucose steady, and I've also noted the snacks that help you get choline too.

→ Make protein a priority in your lunches and dinners. Again, there are recipes for some of my favorite dishes at the end of the book.

→ Find proteins that you like and that you can add to anything. Maybe you love hazelnuts. Maybe you love cottage cheese with capers. Add a handful or a scoop of these to your plate as often as you can.

→ Don't hesitate to keep a **protein powder** in your back pocket to mix into soups or yogurts. You're looking for a whey isolate, unflavored, from grass-fed cows if you eat animal foods; otherwise, a pea and rice protein powder blend. It should contain no sugar, sweeteners, or artificial flavors. Protein powder was my best friend during pregnancy. I had a portion of it every single day in my yogurt snack—page 304. (See my website glucosegoddess.com/pages/best-protein-powders or scan the QR code, right, for my current favorite protein powders depending on the country and dietary requirements.) When it comes to protein drinks, be wary: they are highly processed foods with plenty of additives and either sugar or sweeteners. Best to steer clear. If you want protein on the go, a container of Greek yogurt with no added sugar from the corner shop is a much cleaner way to get a portion.

Protein powders

Try all of these recommendations for a few days, taking note of how much protein you've had each day. You'll get the hang of it quickly and soon it will become second nature.

4. If you can, get someone on protein duty when breastfeeding

Breastfeeding is the moment when your protein needs are highest and where the likelihood of muscle loss is highest too: you need 1.9g of protein per kilogram of bodyweight per day. As you're likely going to feel very tired, it can help to plan some staple meals ahead. Here is what I charged my husband with making for me while I was breastfeeding—I also put the calculations on him so I didn't have to think about any of it.

"What Jessie needs: 133g of protein per day and 550mg+ of choline." A sample of my meals included:

→ Five scrambled eggs on a slice of toasted sourdough, seasoned with a little salt and pepper. Add a side of avocado or herbs for freshness. (35g protein, 500mg+ choline)

→ The Smash Parmesan Patties, recipe on page 294. (58g protein, 160mg choline)

- → Smoked salmon and cream cheese on toast, and a spoonful of fish roe. Finish with a squeeze of lemon. (32g protein, 180mg choline)

- → Pasta mixed with a tomato-based meat sauce made with plenty of minced beef and garlic, topped with a mountain of Parmesan (or less if you aren't a Parmesan addict like me). (45g protein, 90mg choline)

- → Chicken breast cooked in cream with lemon, a side of rice. (40g protein, 90mg choline)

- → Protein shake: frozen berries, 3 scoops of protein powder, almond butter, nuts. (60g protein, 20mg choline)

- → And, of course, all the recipes at the end of this book are great options.

THE RECAP: TO GET ENOUGH PROTEIN DURING PREGNANCY AND BREASTFEEDING

Refer to your calculation on page 156 for your weight in kg.

1st trimester	2nd trimester	3rd trimester	Breastfeeding
Eat what you can depending on your level of nausea. Having some protein snacks may even help ease the nausea. If you aren't nauseous, aim for 1.22g/kg bodyweight per day, but it's okay if you can't stomach any.	Aim for 1.52g/kg bodyweight per day.	Aim for 1.52g/kg bodyweight per day.	Aim for 1.9g/kg bodyweight per day.

→ Have a savory breakfast built around protein

→ When you have a snack, think of protein—a yogurt, or some tofu, or a meaty leftover . . . Also make protein a priority in your lunches and dinners.

→ Find proteins that you like and that you can add to anything. A handful of nuts, a scoop of cottage cheese . . . Whatever calls you.

✸ TOP TIPS ✸

✸ As you reach the last trimester of pregnancy, it might become challenging to eat normal portions of meals as there is less space in your abdomen for your stomach . . . and therefore for food. So focus more and more on protein and choline-rich foods, and less and less on carbohydrates. Protein and choline should take priority over anything sweet, for example.

✶ Your body cannot store extra amino acids. After two days, they get burned for energy if they haven't been used. So you need a continuous flow of new ones every single day.

✶ To help curb nausea, try a little bit of protein, such as a few spoonfuls of yogurt or some nuts, as soon as you wake up.

✶ If you are vegetarian: Focus on eggs and dairy. You can get what you need with those. Add lentils, or other beans, for iron.

✶ If you *are* eating sugar or carbs, consuming them in combination with protein will help lower the corresponding glucose spike, as protein does not raise glucose levels: protein breaks down into amino acids during digestion, not into glucose molecules. When combined with foods that turn to glucose, the protein slows down how quickly the glucose molecules arrive in the bloodstream.

✶ Whenever you're in doubt and you aren't sure what you should eat, go for a protein-rich food. Some hard-boiled eggs with sea salt are a great snack, for example.

Frequently Asked Questions

Can you eat too much protein?
This is a common concern. It's possible, but highly unlikely. The upper safety limit for protein is 3.7g per kilogram of bodyweight per day. Which would be 259g per day for me, so 43 eggs. (That's . . . a lot.) At this point, your kidneys get overworked, your metabolism becomes strained, and it may lead to long-term issues for your baby. But in practice, it's far more common to fall short of your needs than to overshoot them.

What about protein powder?
Check with your care team, but pure protein powder (protein powder as the only ingredient, not mixed with other things such as creatine, and so on) is considered safe during pregnancy. I relied on it heavily by mixing it into my yogurt, but I did my research and used only the protein powder from a source I highly trust. Use this QR code to find my top favorites currently.

Protein powders

What about if I am vegetarian?
In this case focus on eggs and dairy, and plant-based sources of protein.

What about if I am vegan?

If you are vegan, you need to be extra conscientious, and spend time and resources making it work. Watch your iron and B12 intakes like a hawk. Supplement wherever necessary to not fall short on these. Find plant-based sources of protein, and learn about amino acids in depth—see opposite.

Amino acids refresher for vegan diets

You may remember from the beginning of this chapter that there are 20 amino acids. Nine of these are "essential"—**histidine, isoleucine, leucine, lysine, methionine, phenylalanine, threonine, tryptophan, and valine**—meaning you must get them from your diet, because your body cannot make them from within. Just as a car would stall if it were missing a key engine component, your ribosomes will stop being able to work if they don't have access to these nine essential amino acids.

During pregnancy, there's an extra amino acid that becomes essential—arginine—because there's much higher demand for it from the baby. And so, even if you think you're getting "enough" overall protein in grams, if you are not eating enough of all ten of these essential amino acids, your and your baby's ribosomes will be compromised.

Being deficient in essential amino acids during pregnancy leads to growth restriction, is linked to preeclampsia and high blood pressure, and can cause uterine contractions, preterm labor, and premature birth. For example, scientists have shown that when mothers with pregnancies complicated by IUGR are supplemented with arginine, an amino acid that plays a vital role in various bodily functions, birth weight increases by 6.4 percent in babies who were growth restricted, blood pressure reduces in the moms, and babies are less likely to be born prematurely. It shows that if you don't have enough arginine, your baby cannot build the proteins it needs and will effectively stop growing. This is why, if you are vegan, it's absolutely crucial to learn about which amino acids are in which foods, and how to combine them practically and effectively.

Even though some plants contain all 20 amino acids in sufficient quantities (we call them "complete" sources of protein), many plant sources have very little of one or more essential amino acids, which limits their effectiveness as sole protein sources. For example, grains like rice are low in lysine, while legumes such as lentils and beans provide more lysine but are often lower in methionine. So by combining grains with legumes, you'll get all nine essential amino acids in more adequate amounts. Here are the "complete" plant sources of protein, enabling you to get the protein you need without having to consume a lot of extra carbs:

Soy products:

→ Tofu (100g): 8g protein
→ Tempeh (100g): 20g protein
→ Edamame (100g): 11g protein
→ Soy milk: Often contains 7–9g protein per 250mL, although some brands have less—check the label

Vegan protein powders:

→ Rice + Pea protein powder: While rice and peas are incomplete on their own, together they complement each other's amino acid profiles to form a complete protein
→ Soy protein powder: a good option

And here are other "complete" plant sources of protein, but which also come with quite a bit of carbs (**this is the trade-off in vegan diets: you'll need to eat a lot of carbs to get enough protein; or you can rely on protein powder, which is pure protein**):

→ Quinoa (1 cup cooked): 8g protein
→ Amaranth (1 cup cooked): 9g protein
→ Buckwheat (1 cup cooked): 6g protein
→ Sprouted Ezekiel bread (2 slices): 8g protein

Near complete sources of amino acids:

→ Hemp seeds
→ Chia seeds

Choose at least one of each row in the table below every single day to get the amino acids that you need:

Essential Amino Acid	Top Vegan Foods (choose at least one daily)
Lysine	Lentils, chickpeas, black beans, soy (tofu, tempeh, edamame), quinoa
Methionine	Brown rice, oats, buckwheat, millet, amaranth, sesame seeds, Brazil nuts
Leucine, isoleucine, valine	Soy products, pea protein, lentils, pumpkin seeds, hemp seeds
Arginine	Pumpkin seeds, chickpeas, peanuts, sesame seeds, lentils, soy products
Tryptophan, threonine, phenylalanine, histidine	Oats, quinoa, walnuts, hemp seeds, almonds, spirulina

CHAPTER 4
The underwater factor

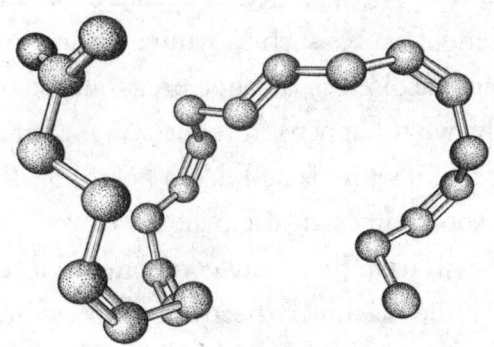

DHA

THE UNDERWATER FACTOR

As we near the end of the book, let's zoom in on your baby's brain. During pregnancy, it is busy creating a staggering **250,000 new neurons per minute.** Next time you brush your teeth, think about this: in these short three minutes, nearly *a million* new brain cells have taken shape inside your womb, built from the raw materials you deliver through the placenta.

In contrast, your adult brain creates about one new neuron per minute. Just *one*. And even that happens only in a tiny corner of the brain, the hippocampus, the seat of memory and learning.

I've said it before: by the time we are born, the majority of our neurons are in place for life. Contrary to other cells in the body, which are on a regular cycle of renewal—some being replaced in a matter of days (gut cells, skin cells), others in decades (bone, muscle)—neurons don't undergo any regeneration: after birth, they just soldier on, without getting replaced, until they die (from a whole variety of causes such as natural ageing, injuries, stroke, neurodegenerative diseases, alcohol, drugs, and so on).

This is why what happens in the womb matters so much: the brain's basic architecture is laid down before birth. By the middle of the second trimester, the majority of your baby's 100 billion neurons will have their core components: a cell membrane, a nucleus, and the machinery needed to process information. By the third trimester, these neurons will be firing and creating the connections that will allow information to travel between them.

So far in this book, we've discussed the impact of steady glucose levels, choline, and protein on the formation of your child's brain. Well, there is another molecule that is critical to its development, and that most babies in utero often don't get enough of. And it comes (mainly) from somewhere you may not expect: *the ocean*. This is the final building block.

Life under the sea

Introducing: **DHA**, short for docosahexaenoic acid. It belongs to the omega-3 family of fats, which includes three main members: ALA, EPA, and DHA. You've probably heard of omega-3s before, as they have a good reputation and are associated with many health benefits. But DHA, in particular, is key.

During pregnancy, molecules of DHA travel from your bloodstream, across the placenta, and into your baby's circulation. Once there, they get to work. DHA helps form the membranes of neurons (alongside choline) and guides their branching arms so they can reach across the brain and link with one another. It helps forge the chemical messengers that allow brain cells to communicate, and it supports the production of BDNF (brain-derived-neurotrophic factor), a molecule that strengthens these connections and underpins learning and memory. DHA also lays down the retina, the delicate sheet of light-sensitive cells at the back of the eye, and with it the rest of the visual system—making it possible for your child to one day observe the world. Not bad for a single nutrient.

As I've said, this vital molecule comes from a surprising place: it is made by **microalgae in the ocean**. That's correct: **your baby's brain formation depends on a molecule produced by microscopic ocean plants.** But don't worry, you don't have to eat the algae itself—you can provide DHA to your fetus by eating DHA-rich animals, which themselves eat microalgae: fish, shellfish, crustaceans. The richest sources are fatty, oily fish such as salmon, sardines, anchovies, mackerel, and herring.

Why did humans develop such a dependency on seafood? The

theory goes like this: About two million years ago, *Homo erectus*, and later *Homo sapiens*, settled near coasts and algae-rich waterways gaining steady access to DHA-rich foods. Pregnant women passed this DHA to their babies, where it fueled rapid brain growth. Many researchers believe this supply of DHA was a key driver of our unusually large brains. Laboratory studies back this up: when scientists grow neurons in dishes and add different fats, only those given DHA nearly double their connections—demonstrating its unique power as a brain "fertilizer."

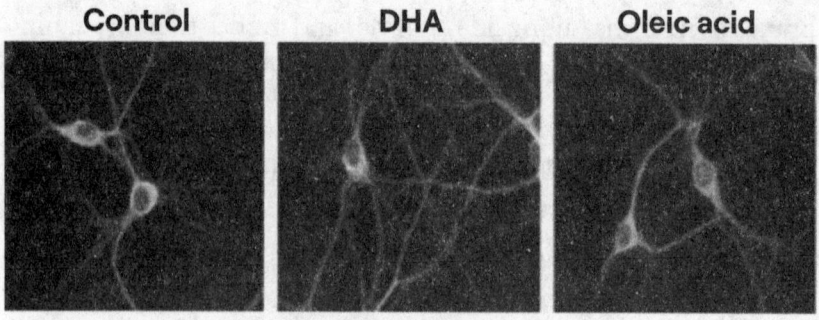

Adapted from Cao et al. 2009

These photos show neurons given different types of fat. The middle photo is the one in which neurons were given DHA. This created nearly double the number of connections between neurons. Other fats in the study made no impact.

So how much DHA do we need? The general consensus among health agencies is that we should get **at least 300mg of DHA per day during pregnancy and breastfeeding** to support our baby's needs and our own. (In the recommendations, it's often phrased as a certain amount of "EPA+DHA," as EPA coexists in foods with DHA. But really, it's the DHA that is most important.)

Unlike protein, DHA is a "slow-build" nutrient that lingers in the body for days after you consume it. This means you don't need to hit exactly 300mg every single day—what matters is your weekly average. To put that into perspective, a daily intake of 300mg is about the same as eating salmon twice a week. (Incidentally, the body *can* make a little DHA on its own—about 20mg per day—and a small fraction of the EPA we eat can be converted into DHA, but the vast majority of our supply has to come directly from food.)

The reality, though, is that most women fall far short: intake is often below 100mg per day, and studies show that **70–95 percent of pregnant women do not reach the 300mg threshold**. This isn't their fault: like the other building blocks in this book, DHA is rarely talked about, and many families face socio-economic barriers to eating fish multiple times a week.

And there's a kicker: 300mg may not be enough. New science shows that there are extra benefits associated with taking much higher doses, of up to 2,200mg (we'll come back to this in a moment). So, what happens if we don't eat enough?

Brains and mazes

Clues about the impact of DHA deficiency can be found in the scientific literature. First, we have **animal studies**. In trials using rats, babies born to mothers who were DHA-deficient during pregnancy and lactation showed measurable cognitive deficits. They struggled to navigate mazes: taking three times as long to reach the exit, making twice as many mistakes, and returning to the wrong path three times more often than their peers. These results matter because maze performance in animals is a standard way to test learning, memory, and problem-solving—skills that, in humans, translate into core aspects of cognitive development.

In studies on monkeys, the animals closest to humans genetically, being born to a DHA-deficient mother led to delays in ocular development, and retinas that had a slower response to light. Even if the offspring were fed a DHA-full diet after birth, their retinas never fully recovered their normal function.

Moving on to humans: first, having low DHA levels could affect the growth of your little one's brain. An MRI study on newborn babies revealed that moms who report eating more omega-3s have babies with larger volumes of frontal cortices and corpus callosum at one month old. These are regions of the brain that manage memory, attention, and communication. It could be that it was the higher amount of DHA available that caused these babies' extra brain growth. A number of observational studies have found that moms with low or no intake of fish during pregnancy have babies born with slower brain responses to what the eyes see, up to 48 percent lower verbal IQ, up to 35 percent reduced fine motor skills, up to 30 percent reduced communication skills, and up to 24 percent reduced social development. In one study from Germany, scientists measured the amount of DHA in the umbilical cord of 400 babies at birth. Then, when the children were ten years old (kudos to the very patient scientists!), they assessed what they called "behavioral difficulties": hyperactivity and inattention in the children. They found that for each 1 percent *increase* in DHA level in the cord blood at birth, the children had a 6 percent *decrease* in these difficulties. The babies with the lowest DHA at birth had nearly twice as many behavioral difficulties as ten-year-olds. Could lacking DHA during development in utero create lasting detriment to a child's brain? Perhaps. But these were just observations.

To parse out the true impact of DHA, scientists have run clinical trials in which they gave pregnant mothers either DHA or a placebo (something that looks like DHA but isn't) during pregnancy. (This is the same study design as the choline-supplementation studies from Chapter 2.) They then measured the differences between the children.

For example, researchers found that when pregnant mothers supplemented with 1,200mg DHA while pregnant, there was a measurable four-point increase in the IQ of their children at four years old. In another study, where pregnant women were given 800mg of DHA per day from week 20 of pregnancy onward, compared to a placebo, significantly fewer children from the DHA group had cognitive scores in the lower range compared with controls (3.1 percent versus 6.4 percent). In yet another study, supplementation of 600mg/day of DHA in the second and third trimesters led to higher levels of sustained attention in infants at four, six, and nine months of age. In an Australian study, pregnant moms received 2.2g (2,200mg) of DHA in the second and third trimesters of pregnancy or a placebo. Their children were assessed at two-and-a-half years old, and those who had received more DHA in the womb had 5.6 percent higher hand-eye coordination scores.

There have been several dozen of these studies, and while some didn't find a measurable difference in the children's outcomes, the ones we just covered revealed striking results. That's not a contradiction: it's how science moves forward. Individual studies give us pieces of the puzzle, and when you put enough of them together, patterns begin to emerge.

Taken together, the evidence tells a powerful story. From rats struggling through mazes, to monkeys with altered vision, to human children scoring higher on IQ tests or showing fewer behavioral difficulties . . . The amount of DHA available in the womb as your baby grows and connects his neurons can shape his brain in ways that echo years later. And good news: as you'll learn in the Action Plan, it's easy for you to up your intake significantly (even if you don't eat fish, I've got options for you).

That said, boosting DHA is only half the story. To truly give your baby the best chance, there's another substance you need to dial down at the same time—one that works in opposition to omega-3s. That's what we'll learn about now.

The cervix and omega-6

Just like any good movie, the world of omegas has its heroes and antiheroes. On the hero side are the omega-3s, such as DHA. Not only do omega-3s build your baby's brain, they also play a key role in *calming inflammation.*

On the other side sit the omega-6s. They *encourage inflammation.* They aren't evil, as we need them for things like blood clotting and healthy cell structure. But the plot twist comes when they aren't in balance: when omega-6s overwhelm omega-3s, the body tilts toward excess and detrimental inflammation. This is when trouble begins.

The way we assess the state of our omega levels is via something called the **omega-6 to omega-3 ratio**. In the 1900s, this ratio in most people's diets was about 3:1. Which meant we ate about three times as many omega-6s as we did omega-3s. A manageable balance. But in modern Western diets, the ratio can be up to **20:1**. This means that we have much higher levels of omega-6s than before, therefore more inflammation in the body than we used to.

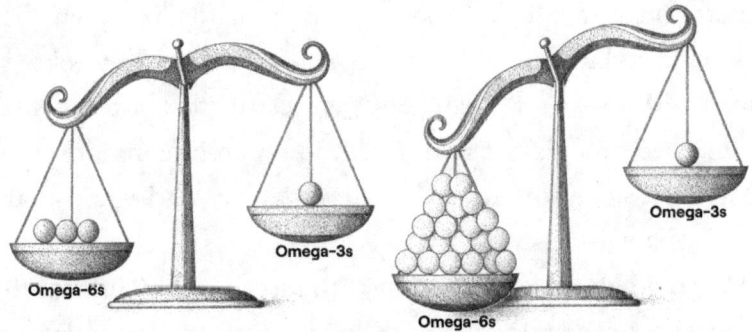

In the 1900s, humans had about three times more omega-6s in their blood than omega-3s. Today, we have about 20 times more omega-6s than omega-3s. This gets transferred to your baby and leads to higher inflammation levels.

Omega-3s and small quantities of omega-6s usually come packaged together in foods like nuts, seeds, eggs, and fish. But in the past few decades, our diets have shifted dramatically and omega-6 fats have taken over. Processed oils such as soybean, sunflower, corn, and cottonseed now dominate the food supply: they are *packed with omega-6s*, and contain virtually zero omega-3s. These oils show up in dressings, chips, baked goods, frozen meals, and fried fast food, making omega-6s almost impossible to avoid. At the same time, foods rich in omega-3s, such as fish, seaweed, grass-fed dairy and beef, and free-range, pasture-raised eggs, are eaten far less often. As a result, keeping omega-3s and omega-6s in balance has become almost impossible.

As we saw in Chapter 1, high levels of inflammation can disrupt fetal development. But here's what's interesting: labor and birth are themselves triggered by inflammation. **To soften the cervix and start contractions, your body produces inflammatory molecules made from omega-6 fats called prostaglandins.** It's a powerful, natural mechanism, and one that doctors sometimes mimic when inducing labor (see page 239 for labor tips).

The problem comes when this system switches on too early. Preterm birth rates in the US have risen nearly 30 percent since 1980, and today one in ten babies is born before 37 weeks (full term is 40 weeks). Researchers suspect that our excess intake of omega-6 fats plays a role here: **too much inflammation may cause prostaglandins to activate prematurely, triggering labor before a baby is ready.**

When a baby is born too early, he misses out on critical time in the womb when organs are still maturing. The last four weeks of pregnancy are especially important: **more DHA is transferred to the baby during this window than in all the previous weeks**

combined. While many preterm babies do fine (I was born at 36 weeks; hi there), preterm birth remains a leading cause of disability and death in the first five years of life, and raises the risk of developing long-term health conditions such as heart disease. Babies born at 34–36 weeks have a 30 percent increased risk of neurodevelopmental impairments (such as motor, cognitive, epileptic, visual, or hearing impairments) and a 38 percent higher risk of lower cognitive ability compared to full-term peers. Even those born "early term" (at 37–38 weeks) score, on average, three IQ points lower, with each extra week in the womb improving cognitive scores. They also have slightly reduced problem-solving skills and higher rates of ADHD. Across studies, being born before 37 weeks is linked to 5 percent lower cognitive performance, a 30–50 percent greater likelihood of needing special education, and lower achievement in math and reading. It should be said that these are all associative studies and **the absolute risks remain low—most babies born a little early do very well. But still, every extra week in the womb offers a small but meaningful boost for long-term health and development.**

So, the question is: Can we tip the scales back in the baby's favor? Can increasing our omega-3 intake and lowering inflammation help prevent labor from starting too soon? Remarkably, the science suggests the answer is yes.

To test this simple but very powerful idea, scientists have run clinical trials supplementing thousands of pregnant moms with omega 3s. The results are unequivocal: **taking omega-3s during pregnancy successfully reduces the risk of preterm births.** In the studies, those who supplemented with omega-3s or focused on getting enough omega-3s through food reduced the risk of their baby being born before 34 weeks from 4.6 percent to 2.7 percent.

Similarly, the risk of giving birth before 37 weeks reduced from 13.4 percent to 11.9 percent. An incredible discovery.

And it isn't just supplements. Across tens of thousands of women worldwide, eating fish during pregnancy has consistently been linked with lower rates of preterm birth and better long-term outcomes for children. The evidence is strong enough for some countries (for example, Australia) to now be recommending 800–1,000mg of DHA per day for women at risk of preterm birth, well above the standard 200–500mg.

Nor do the benefits of calming inflammation stop at reducing the risk of preterm birth: as you may remember from Chapter 1, lower inflammation during pregnancy is not only linked to healthier development, but also to a reduced risk of neurodevelopmental disorders later on.

Taken together, the evidence is crystal clear: DHA is a must-have for your baby's development and lifelong health. And yet so few of us are getting enough. Those figures showing that 70–95 percent of moms are deficient really struck me. I wanted to know where I stood.

Eight percent

During my pregnancy, the scientist in me couldn't resist getting my blood drawn regularly. (Was my husband slightly concerned I was having an affair with my phlebotomist? Perhaps.) But I just *had* to see what was happening in my body, by testing my own levels of inflammation and omegas.

So let's get to some numbers. First, **inflammation.** As we saw in Chapter 1, the most common way to measure inflammation is with a simple blood test called the C-reactive protein (CRP) test. I was at 0.7mg/L prepregnancy, and 1.7mg/L at six months pregnant. It's normal for inflammation in your body to increase as pregnancy progresses. But too much of it can have consequences. Remaining on the lower end is better, as studies show that levels of CRP above 8mg/L start to be associated with a higher risk of preterm delivery. To reduce inflammation, we have several levers we can pull: we can ensure we have a proper intake of omega-3s, we can try to decrease our omega-6s, and we can manage our starches and sugars to reduce our glucose spikes (more on all of this in the Action Plan at the end of the chapter).

Second, **omega-3s.** A robust way to check whether you have enough omega-3s is to run a blood test called the **omega-3 index** (if you do, make sure it's done by looking at the red blood cell index, not the plasma index, as the red blood cell one is representative of long-term intake). The omega-3 index measures how many omega-3s are integrated into your blood-cell membranes, as a proportion of the overall omegas. This test is truly the best measure of overall omega-3 health in your body. **An important goal during pregnancy is getting your omega-3 index above**

8 percent. Below 4 percent means you are in an omega-3 deficit; mid-range is 5–8 percent, and optimal is 8–12 percent (it's very rare to be above 12 percent, but it is even better).

If you want to run this test, check whether your insurance covers it, because it can be very expensive ($200 or more, as an estimate). But whether you test or not, you can be pretty sure you're below the desired level. **In a study of 250 pregnant women, only 4 percent had an omega-3 index superior to the recommended 8 percent.** *Four percent.* But perhaps this is not so surprising: recent international studies have shown that you actually need about 2,000mg EPA+DHA daily for three months to get your levels up from 4 percent to 8 percent. This is much higher than the generic 300mg or more recommendation.

So, what to do? Ideally, you need to get at least the recommended 300mg a day of DHA, but up to 2,000mg daily might be what is needed depending on your omega-3 index level. In the Action Plan at the end of this chapter, I'll go over supplements that you may want to check out if you want to go up to 2,000mg.

Personally, I went even higher. Here's my data: Two years before trying to conceive ("TTC" on the graph), I checked my omega-3 index. It was good but not optimal: 6.8 percent. So I started eating salmon once a week and took an omega-3 supplement (which contained 750mg EPA and 510mg DHA, which is about the equivalent of eating an extra serving of salmon every day). A year later, I had got it up to 7.9 percent. I then doubled my omega-3 supplements to two doses per day (for a total of 1,020mg DHA per day). Six months later, just before my first pregnancy, I was at 11.3 percent.

At seven months pregnant, and despite continuing my routine of supplementing with 1,020mg DHA daily, and eating fatty fish three times a week now, it had dropped to 8.6 percent.

This is normal because of the large transfer of DHA to my baby, but I was thrilled to see that I was still above the ideal 8 percent this far into my pregnancy. This meant my baby was getting all the DHA he needed.

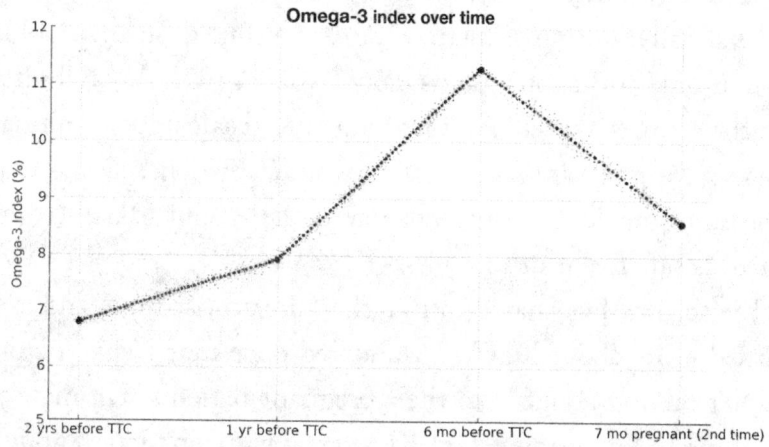

My omega-3 index over time, which I increased thanks to eating more salmon and taking omega-3 supplements. It decreased during my pregnancy despite the same routine (and even more supplements), showing the large transfer to my baby.

And, if you have gestational diabetes, here is another reason to up your omega-3s: in trials on moms with a gestational-diabetes diagnosis, taking an omega-3 supplement was shown to significantly reduce fasting glucose levels by 4.5mg/dL. In these moms, the omega-3 supplementation also reduced their CRP levels.

During breastfeeding, the transfer of DHA continues in large quantities. But how much depends on your index. For example, the results of one study show that when a breastfeeding mom takes a supplement of 400mg of DHA, her breast milk contains **twice as much DHA** as that of a mom who doesn't take the supplement. This is why you'll find DHA in virtually all baby formula: it's essential to a newborn's brain. The recommended daily amount during breastfeeding is similar to that in pregnancy—that is at least **300mg per day**. It's important to continue providing DHA for your baby at this stage, and for up to two years of life. After this window, the connections in the brain are largely set, and it becomes much harder to reshape.

Personally, during breastfeeding, I continued on my double dose of omega-3 supplements daily (1,020mg DHA), and fatty fish three times a week. Although no official safe upper limit has been set for pregnant and lactating women, evidence shows that consuming up to 5,000mg per day of EPA and DHA (combined) is safe for healthy adults.

The science I've shared in this chapter surprised me, and as I learned more about DHA, I wondered once more why doctors weren't talking about it to their pregnant patients. Ultimately, the thing to know about DHA is that, if you don't have enough of it, your baby will not get what he needs either, because your body must keep some stores for you to maintain brain function. This has been demonstrated by scientists, who have measured the DHA levels in the umbilical cord of babies at birth, and found that these vary widely, depending on the mom's concentrations.

Just as with the other building blocks (glucose, choline, and protein)—indeed with most nutrients—the amount of omega-3 you eat will be reflected in your baby's own circulation: **If you eat less DHA during pregnancy, your baby will get less. If you eat more, your baby will get more.** This is yet further proof that the idea that "your baby will get what he needs from you" regardless of your diet is a fallacy.

Pass the peanuts

It turns out that DHA can also help mitigate against the development of allergies in our babies. Allergic reactions (asthma, eczema, food allergies, and so on) are an overactive response of the immune system to harmless substances. And fascinating new research shows that you can potentially shape your baby's long-term risk of these while he is in the womb. Your baby's immune system starts to develop during pregnancy, and mothers who have higher amounts of anti-inflammatory omega-3s during this time can help prevent it from overreacting. When you keep your inflammation low during pregnancy, you also create a low-inflammation environment in your baby's body, which encourages healthy immune responses—not overactive ones.

In a large study that looked at 3,000 moms and their children, supplementing with omega-3s during pregnancy and breastfeeding reduced the risk of eczema in toddlers by 39 percent. In another landmark trial, pregnant women who took 2,400mg of DHA- and EPA-rich fish oil daily during the third trimester cut their child's risk of asthma by nearly one-third: 16.9 percent of children developed asthma or persistent wheeze, compared to 23.7 percent in the placebo group.

A further study found maternal omega-3 supplementation during pregnancy reduced the risk of any food allergy by 47 percent, egg allergy by 42 percent, and peanut allergy by 38 percent in offspring. If the children themselves were given supplements after birth, there was no effect—the reductions happened only when a mom supplemented while pregnant, suggesting that the omega-3 levels in the mom tilted the baby's immune system in utero away from over-reacting. This is such an interesting and powerful insight.

High sugar and high carbohydrate intake during pregnancy are also linked to impaired lung development in the fetus, slightly increasing the child's risk of respiratory infections, asthma, allergies, and even certain cancers later in life. A study found that **children of mothers with the highest sugar intake (more than 80g per day, which is what most people consume on a daily basis today) had a 38 percent higher risk of allergies and are more than twice as likely to develop allergic asthma, independent of their further sugar intake in childhood.** Scientists believe this is owing to sugar-induced inflammation in the developing lungs, and animal studies suggest that reducing inflammation through a high-fiber maternal diet can lower the risk of asthma, reinforcing the idea that asthma may begin before birth.

On the topic of food allergies, we used to believe that in order to prevent them, we should not eat allergy-prone foods during pregnancy—but we now know this isn't true, and could even backfire. In fact, some observational studies suggest that maternal consumption of allergenic foods (such as peanuts, tree nuts, and so on), rather than increasing allergy risk in children, might promote tolerance—although introducing them in an infant's diet plays a larger role. Additionally, antioxidants from fruits and vegetables in a mom's diet can help shape a robust immune system in the fetus.

Seaweed and pickles

But back to where DHA comes from: the ocean. DHA isn't the only aquatic treasure that matters for your baby's lifelong health. There's another mineral, also found underwater, that quietly shapes the brain: **iodine**.

Iodine is essential for making thyroid hormones, which regulate your baby's brain and nervous system development. During pregnancy, your iodine need climbs by about 50 percent to 250mcg per day. But guess what: from food intake alone, **only 47 percent of pregnant women get enough of it.**

The consequences can range from lower IQ scores in children in the case of moderate deficiency, all the way to cretinism in the case of severe deficiency, one of the most devastating and preventable causes of intellectual disability. Controlled trials in iodine-deficient regions confirm that supplementing mothers during pregnancy improves their children's developmental scores.

The good news is that it doesn't take much to meet your 250mcg-per-day iodine goal if you know to focus on it: many prenatal supplements contain some iodine; it's often added to salt (check on the label whether your salt is iodized); and it's easy to get enough from food: fish and shellfish are rich sources of iodine, because they get it from the algae they eat. Seaweed is a powerful source: one nori sheet (2.8g) contains about 100mcg. But iodine isn't just found in the sea—as water evaporates and rain falls, it makes its way into the soil too. And from there, it trickles into our drinking water, into our fruits and vegetables, and, in higher amounts, into foods like milk, eggs, and even meat. Dairy is the second-best source of iodine after seafood, with 115mcg in 250g of Greek yogurt and 60mcg in a standard mozzarella ball. Eggs contribute around 25mcg each. **This means that four eggs and a large portion of Greek yogurt get you roughly to the 250mcg-per-day target.** Or, add some nori sheets to your meal prep: during my pregnancy I often cut them into squares and dropped them into soup or lentils, since I have never liked chewing them raw. If you use iodized salt, it's even easier to reach your goal.

While getting enough iodine is crucial, it's also important not to go overboard. Health authorities have set a recommended upper limit of 1,100mcg per day during pregnancy and lactation (equivalent to eating 11 nori sheets per day), as high intakes may disrupt thyroid function (in both moms and babies) by temporarily suppressing thyroid hormone production. This is especially a concern for women who already have thyroid disease or autoimmunity, as their thyroids are more sensitive to big iodine swings.

One final underwater treasure we must discuss: salt. **You know those classic pickle or salty foods cravings?** They actually be your body asking for salt. Salt is essential for blood volume, electrolyte balance, and fetal growth. Contrary to popular belief, salt does not cause pregnancy water retention or hypertension in most women. In fact, low salt intake has been linked to higher risks of intrauterine growth restriction, preterm birth, and poor blood sugar control. Salting your food is totally fine, but you can go overboard if you have too much (more than 10g per day, for example; or two teaspoons), especially if you already have high blood pressure or are at high risk of preeclampsia. But for most healthy pregnancies, there's no clear benefit to cutting salt. Think of it, like iodine itself, as another underwater treasure that helps your baby's brain and body grow strong.

ACTION PLAN

Time to review DHA and iodine. First, let's get practical with DHA, our fourth and final pregnancy building block. Just as with choline, we've got a general lower-end recommendation (300mg DHA daily), but measurable benefits in studies at much higher doses (up to 2,200mg DHA per day).

The exact target is something to decide with your care team. But if you're already well into pregnancy and haven't focused on DHA before, or if your omega-3 index is low, it can make sense to aim higher. Personally, I averaged around 1,520mg of DHA per day (1,020mg of DHA daily from the supplement I took, plus fatty fish three times a week, which adds an extra 500mg DHA per day). Even at that intake, my omega-3 index dropped significantly during pregnancy—but I was able to stay above my 8 percent goal.

For this Action Plan, I'm setting 500mg of DHA per day as the target. It's a realistic lower-end goal, above the baseline recommendation. For iodine, the general recommendation of 250mcg is our goal. Let's look at these each in turn.

1. Eat oily fish three times a week, starting as soon as possible

Start early. **DHA takes time to build up in your body.** Unlike protein, which you use and clear daily, DHA is a "slow-build" nutrient. Your body tucks it into cell membranes and gradually amasses reserves, so by the third trimester (when your baby's brain and eyes are growing at full speed), you can release a steady supply across the placenta. That's why it's recommended to begin DHA-rich foods as soon as possible, even preconception, to build up your stores.

Think in weekly totals. You don't have to eat DHA every single day, as long as your weekly average adds up. So, **aim for roughly 3,500mg across the week,** to average out at 500mg per day. A practical way to hit this is to eat salmon, sardines, anchovies, trout, or herring about three times per week. (The standard advice is twice weekly; three gives you a better margin.) Oily saltwater fish are the richest DHA sources. Most freshwater fish have less DHA because they don't feed on marine microalgae (the original source) and depend on converting plant fats.

To get to your goal choose three servings of approximately 100g fish per week:

→ Salmon: 1,460mg DHA per serving
→ Anchovy: 1,200mg DHA
→ Herring: 1,100mg DHA
→ Sardines: 870mg DHA
→ Mackerel: 690mg DHA

Also helpful but with less DHA (per 100g portion):

→ Sea bass: 470mg DHA
→ Trout: 440mg DHA
→ Haddock: 110mg DHA
→ Carp: 150mg DHA
→ Catfish: 50mg DHA
→ Tuna: 170mg DHA
→ Tilapia: 50mg DHA
→ Perch/Pike/Bass: about 50–100mg DHA

At the end of this book, you'll find delicious recipes to incorporate fish easily into your weekly meal plan.

→ **A DHA bonus from eggs:** Free-range, pasture-raised eggs contain 30mg of DHA each. That's because the hens eat grass, bugs, and feed rich in omega-3s. Standard supermarket eggs often contain little to none. So if you're eating four free-range pasture-raised eggs a day for your choline needs, you'll also be getting an extra 120mg of DHA without lifting a finger. Look for "pasture-raised" or "omega-3 enriched" on the packaging.

What about mercury in fish? Research shows that the health benefits of consuming seafood during the prenatal period outweigh the potential risks. But you can err on the side of caution and skip tuna, which is a high-mercury fish, if you prefer.

During breastfeeding, try to get the same amount. That's **3,500mg across the week,** to average out at 500mg per day. You can use the same servings of fish as during pregnancy, and you can also add in new foods that aren't recommended during pregnancy because of potential infections, but are okay when breastfeeding:

→ Sushi/sashimi/poke/tartare
→ Cold-smoked or cured fish: lox, gravlax, cold-smoked mackerel, cold-smoked herring/kippers
→ Ceviche (citrus or vinegar-cured raw fish)
→ Raw shellfish: oysters, clams, mussels (fresh, from a reputable source)
→ Salt-cured roe beyond caviar: bottarga, taramasalata (roe spread)

2. Learn about supplements that could support you

If you eat oily fish three times a week, you'll reach about 500mg of DHA per day: the daily goal of this Action Plan. But as you saw in the omega-3 index study I mentioned earlier, higher intakes may be even better if your aim is to get your index above 8 percent. To increase your levels, you can either eat more fish or add an omega-3 supplement.

Most general prenatal supplements don't include omega-3s. They're usually left out because omega-3s are bulky, expensive, and sensitive to heat. That means if you want them, you'll need to look for a separate omega-3 supplement. The exact amount you take is up to you.

Omega-3 supplements always come as a combination of EPA and DHA (although be aware that while EPA has its own benefits, it converts very poorly into DHA, and DHA is the one that matters most for your baby's brain). For example, the supplement I took contained 750mg of EPA and 510mg of DHA per dose. During pregnancy, I doubled that to two doses a day, giving me just over 1,000mg of DHA. When making your selection, you've got a few big things to look out for:

→ **Concentration:** Look in the nutrition facts and check how much DHA specifically is in each serving. Many supplements called "Omega-3 supplements" will contain a lot of EPA and little DHA. But now you know that what you actually need is DHA. Look for at least 500mg of DHA per serving.

→ **Form:** Omega-3 supplements don't all come in the same chemical package. They can be in triglyceride form (the way they naturally appear in fish), in ethyl ester form (a cheaper, processed version) or in phospholipid form (like in krill oil). Your body absorbs them best in the triglyceride or phospholipid forms, while the ethyl ester form is less well absorbed.

→ **Toxicity and oxidation:** Because fish can accumulate mercury and other pollutants, it's important to choose supplements that are third-party tested for heavy metals and contaminants. Omega-3 fats are also fragile: they oxidize easily when exposed to heat, light or air. Oxidized oils not only lose their benefits but may even be harmful. That's why you should look for **omega-3 supplements that come in dark capsules or bottles.**

As a reminder, I took 1,020mg of DHA supplements per day during pregnancy and while breastfeeding. But you should determine your intake with your provider, based on your omega-3 index if you have access to that number.

We saw a lot of studies earlier showing how omega-3 supplementation during pregnancy mitigates against preterm birth. I should say here that there is a potential caveat to this: some studies have shown that **supplementing with very large doses of omega-3s in the final weeks of pregnancy can actually increase the length of gestation, and potentially push mothers to go over term** (although the strength of this evidence is weaker). Ask your care team whether they advise stopping supplements in the last month of pregnancy. Personally, in the ninth month, I stopped the supplements and focused on salmon. And then, as soon as I gave birth, I started back on the supplements.

If you are vegan or don't eat fish, find an algae-based omega-3 supplement. This is essential—don't skip it.

Check my website for my top picks for omega-3 supplements that are ideal in terms of concentration and form, and with low toxicity and oxidation: glucosegoddess.com/pages/supplements-pregnancy

My top omega-3 supplements

3. Get some iodine

Your goal during pregnancy and breastfeeding is to consume **at least 250mcg of iodine** per day, up from 150mcg per day when not pregnant. If you use iodized salt at each meal, you're already covering a big part of your iodine needs. A single gram of iodized salt contains about 45mcg of iodine, so if you're salting food normally throughout the day, you'll likely reach about 4g total. That's roughly 135–180mcg of iodine. However, not all salts are iodized: standard table salt often is; most sea salts, Himalayan pink salt, and fancy finishing salts usually are not. Look for "iodized" on the label. I also added nori sheets a couple of times a week to my snacks and meals to make sure I was getting enough.

If you consume fish three times a week which is recommended for omega-3 intake, you will also get iodine from them:

→ Haddock portion: 420mcg (the only fish with very high iodine is haddock)
→ One portion of salmon, herring, anchovies, sardines, or other fish: average 20–60mcg

Dairy is also a great source of iodine, and it contains great quantities of protein too:

→ 250g of Greek yogurt: 115mcg
→ 250ml of milk: 85mcg

Additional foods that will help you get to 250mcg daily:

→ Langoustine: 300mcg per portion
→ Crab: 225mcg per portion
→ Nori sheet: 100mcg each
→ An egg: 25mcg

The safe upper limit of iodine is 1,100mcg per day, or 7,700mcg weekly. At the end of this book, you'll find delicious recipes that feature nori and yogurt to help you reach your iodine goals.

4. Continue during breastfeeding, or pick the right formula

During breastfeeding, the recommendation for DHA is similar, because your baby's brain is still highly dependent on this building block after birth. If your baby is formula-fed, it's crucial that his formula contains DHA. You can check this by looking at the Nutritional Facts on the back of the package. For a long time DHA was not added to formula, and it still isn't a mandatory ingredient in most countries. In Europe, it became mandatory in 2021. Studies show that DHA-enriched formula leads to measurably better development, with infants scoring higher on cognitive tests compared to those on standard formula.

5. Reduce omega-6s in your life

As we saw earlier, the real issue with omega-6s today is the overwhelming quantities hidden in industrial oils—like soybean, corn, sunflower, and safflower—that saturate modern cooking and food manufacturing. These oils are everywhere, and they push our omega-6 levels far too high.

They also happen to be a cornerstone of ultra-processed foods, which are often loaded with sugar as well. And as you learned in Chapter 1, too much sugar in pregnancy can harm your baby. The good news? By cutting back on processed foods to lower your intake of omega-6-rich oils, you'll also automatically cut back on sugar. Add in the Chapter 1 hacks, and those cravings will lose their grip over time.

THE RECAP: TO GET ENOUGH DHA AND IODINE DURING PREGNANCY AND BREASTFEEDING

1st trimester	2nd trimester	3rd trimester	Breastfeeding
Supplement with omega-3s if you can stomach them	Supplement with omega-3s	Supplement with omega-3s, but potentially stop supplements a little bit before the due date, depending on the advice of your care team	Supplement with omega-3s
Eat fish 3x week if you can (even 1 portion is good, so don't worry if 3 is a struggle)	Eat fish 3x week if you can	Eat fish 3x week if you can	Eat fish 3x week if you can
~250mcg/day of iodine, in salt, supplement, or nori	~250mcg/day of iodine	~250mcg/day of iodine	~250mcg/day of iodine

→ Eat oily fish three times a week, starting as early as possible.

→ Consider supplementing with omega-3s.

→ Add iodized salt, nori sheets, or dairy to get iodine.

★ TOP TIPS ★

★ Don't delay. If you've been topping up your "DHA savings account" from the start of your pregnancy, you'll have more to give when demand peaks. Waiting until the third trimester means playing catch-up.

* Wild-caught salmon is ideal, but even farm-raised salmon contains high levels of DHA (sometimes even higher, since many farms now add algae oil to boost omega-3s).

* Fish is a great protein source—so you will also be getting your protein in!

* If you eat eggs, choose free-range, pasture-raised eggs if you can. They naturally contain 30mg of DHA each. Standard supermarket eggs do not contain DHA (but if you eat those, it's completely okay—they still contain choline and protein).

Frequently Asked Questions

Instead of fish can I get DHA directly from algae?
Yes, you can! This is the best option for vegans to meet DHA needs. You can find algae-based supplements or algae oil.

Can I rely on my body making its own DHA from plant sources?
We can make a little DHA from ALA (alpha-linolenic acid), an omega-3 found in seeds like flax and chia. But the conversion is very inefficient: usually less than 5 percent, and often closer to 1–2 percent during pregnancy. The conversion rate also depends on your genes, sex, and how much omega-6 you eat (a high omega-6 diet makes conversion even weaker). During

pregnancy, the demand for DHA often outpaces the conversion capacity. So trying to compensate for this deficiency through plant sources is an uphill struggle: where 100g of salmon provides about 1,500mg of DHA, to get the same amount just from flaxseed oil, you'd need to consume 42 tablespoons every single day. That's over 600ml of oil. Intense.

In summary: while plant sources of ALA are healthy and worth including, you cannot rely upon them to meet your DHA needs in pregnancy. Direct sources like fish, algae oil, or supplements are the only reliable way to ensure your baby gets enough. Dietary DHA is also the most efficient form: it bypasses the need for conversion and is incorporated straight into cell membranes, especially in the brain and retina, where your baby needs it most.

Our ancestors didn't always have fish, so surely we must have evolved to make enough DHA from plants?
This is evolutionarily plausible but known not to be optimal today. While our ancestors—who didn't have access to fish—could survive on the plant-based omega-3 conversion, it doesn't mean it was ideal for thriving.

All animal brains need DHA—but most animals don't eat fish. How is this possible?
All animals need DHA in their brains, but most require only small amounts because their brains are much smaller than ours. For them, the limited DHA made from plant-based omega-3s is often enough.

CHAPTER 5

The final crumbs

EXERCISE, ALCOHOL, COFFEE & TEA,
FRUIT & VEG, FERMENTED FOODS, PLASTIC

THE FINAL CRUMBS

In the previous chapters, we've covered what I consider to be the four major building blocks of pregnancy nutrition: managing glucose levels, and loading up on choline, protein, and DHA. In this final chapter, I'll tackle a few extra topics that I wondered about myself during my pregnancy. I went looking for answers, and I've shared them with you here.

Exercise

I'll state the obvious: exercise makes us feel better, both physically and mentally. And these days, moms are increasingly being encouraged by health professionals to maintain some kind of exercise regime while they are pregnant. Which is great news. I exercised throughout my pregnancy (mostly lifting weights and walking to and from the gym) and honestly, it kept me sane. But . . . little-known fact: exercising during pregnancy can actually nurture your *baby's* mental health too.

A fascinating study from Dokuz Eylül University in Turkey tested this idea in an unusual way. Researchers divided pregnant rats into two groups. One group walked on a tiny little treadmill for 30 minutes a day, five days a week, throughout pregnancy. The other group stayed sedentary. Everything else (diet, light, housing) was kept exactly the same.

The results were striking. The babies born to the moms who exercised solved maze puzzles about 1.5 times more efficiently, made 60 percent fewer errors and—once they grew up—their hippocampus (the brain's learning and memory hub) was more developed. They had 20 percent more neurons across key memory regions of the brain, learned 40 percent faster, and showed 80 percent lower levels of anxiety.

So what was happening? Exercise triggers the production of a remarkable molecule in the hippocampus called BDNF, short for brain-derived neurotrophic factor (I mentioned it briefly in the previous chapter). BDNF helps the brain to grow new neurons, strengthen connections, and adapt. Low levels of BDNF are linked to aggressive behavior, anxiety, and a higher risk of depression or bipolar disorder. When you exercise, whether during pregnancy or not, your brain produces BDNF. It's one of the reasons that exercise is great for our mental health.

In the Turkish study, the scientists measured BDNF levels directly. As expected, the pregnant rats who exercised had higher BDNF in their brains compared to the sedentary ones. But here's the fascinating part: their babies did too. The offspring of the active moms showed higher BDNF levels than the offspring of the non-exercising moms—and this boost didn't fade. It carried through the offsprings' childhood and remained into adulthood. **This increased BDNF could explain the benefits on the pups' cognition and mental health.**

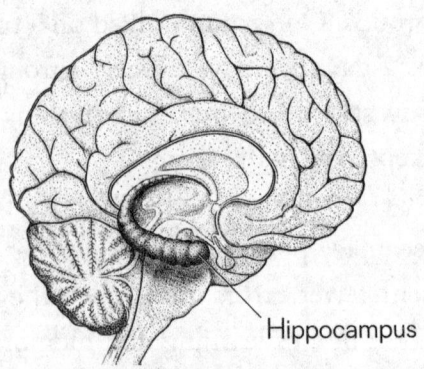

Was the mom's BDNF simply crossing the placenta? We don't know for sure yet—but it may be even cooler than that. Scientists think that exercise during pregnancy may flip epigenetic switches in the baby's DNA, programming their own brain to make more BDNF.

The conclusion of this research is that **exercising during pregnancy may gift your baby a hidden superpower—a brain richer**

in BDNF, packed with more neurons, and more adaptable for life. And remember: by the time your baby is born, most of those neurons are already in place. So whether it's getting enough choline, cutting back on sugar to reduce inflammation, or staying active, every choice helps lay down the lifelong foundation of your child's brain.

It might be worth busting a few popular myths here: despite what you may have heard, exercising during pregnancy does not reduce blood flow to the baby (there is no scientific evidence behind this whatsoever), nor does it reduce the baby's heart rate. There actually seems to be *more* blood flow to your baby after exercise, and a reduction in inflammation too. But old beliefs die hard: surveys show that about half of doctors in the US still tell their pregnant patients to limit exercises that increase heart rate during pregnancy.

We have a few human studies that also point to benefits. In one study from Brazil, 420 moms were split into two groups at random. One group was asked to exercise three times a week in the second half of their pregnancy, while the other group was asked not to. The study found that children of the mothers who were asked to exercise during pregnancy had slightly higher language scores at age two and cognitive scores at age four.

Continuing regular exercise throughout pregnancy is also correlated to babies having about 7 percent better early motor skills at one year old, and improved performance on general intelligence (about 8 percent better) and oral language skills (about 9 percent better) at five years old. And here are some more motivating associations: babies born to women who combined aerobic and resistance training during pregnancy have been shown to be more alert, better at self-soothing, and less agitated. In another study, kids born to moms who lifted weights during pregnancy were more attentive, as well as more cognitively advanced than their peers. Of course, these are again just associations—the animal studies are more revealing as they are controlled.

Finally, there are benefits to you too. During pregnancy, physical function—measured as the ability to perform normal daily activities—declines from 95 percent to 58 percent in the third trimester, and prevalence of depression increases from 11 percent prior to pregnancy to 25 percent during that same time. Regular exercise and resistance training reduces fatigue, increases physical and mental energy, reduces bleeding after birth, reduces complications during birth, and reduces back pain throughout. It also reduces the risk of gestational diabetes by *half* (!), as well as complications from it if a mother already has it; it reduces the likelihood of a baby being born too big, helps your body manage glucose levels better, which allows your baby to grow in a healthier womb environment, and in some studies increases vaginal deliveries and reduces C-sections. Exercising is also linked to a more muscular body composition postpartum. So . . . a lot!

And here's something cool: exercising while pregnant is the equivalent of training at high altitude like professional athletes do. (This is why tackling any small hill during pregnancy will feel like climbing Mount Everest.) When you're pregnant, your body naturally increases blood volume and heart rate, while your growing uterus slightly reduces your lung capacity—together, this creates a state where oxygen delivery is less efficient. Just as with altitude training, your pregnant body adapts by boosting red blood cells and improving circulation, and is forced to become more efficient at delivering oxygen. All of which upgrades your cardiovascular system: more red blood cells, a more efficient heart. Once you're postpartum, your body retains some of those adaptations for a little while and keeps you cardiovascularly fitter. Fancy altitude training, for free.

As for the question of whether exercise during pregnancy can help with the birthing experience, some studies have found that it has no impact, and does not change the length of labor, while other studies have found that it helps reduce women's labor time.

So as long as your doctor has cleared it, go for a walk or pick up some weights. Or get on a treadmill and walk just like the rat moms did. Whatever you feel like. The best exercise is the one that you're going to do. The World Health Organization recommends 150 minutes per week of moderate physical activity during pregnancy. **Yet only 23 percent of pregnant women get that amount,** based on a US survey. I'm sure that number would be higher if everyone knew about this science.

Alcohol

For decades, we were told that "a glass of wine a day is good for the heart." Growing up in France, this idea was practically served as fact alongside a baguette. But modern science has overturned it.

The previous studies that suggested there were benefits from moderate drinking were flawed: the "non-drinker" groups in those studies often included people who had quit alcohol because of health problems. That made the abstainers look less healthy, while the moderate drinkers, who hadn't yet developed disease, appeared to fare better. This statistical illusion came to be known as the "sick quitter effect."

When researchers corrected for this bias, the supposed heart-protective effect of alcohol vanished. And more recent large-scale studies and meta-analyses have found no safe threshold for drinking at all. Even small amounts carry measurable downsides. For example, a 2022 analysis of nearly 37,000 people found that consuming just one drink per day was associated with damage to their brain wiring and reductions in their total brain volume—meaning brain cells were shrinking or even dying. As you can imagine, alcohol—being a neurotoxin—is not good for your baby's brain either.

Now, do you remember from Chapter 1 what we learned about the placenta? That your placenta is not a strict bouncer, and what is in your bloodstream will be reflected in your baby's bloodstream from the second trimester onward? Alcohol is no exception. It crosses the placenta freely and, as your own blood-alcohol concentration rises after drinking, so does your baby's in parallel.

Would you think it's a good idea to give your newborn baby a glass of red wine? Probably not. And yet that's essentially what's happening every time you drink one while he's in the womb.

This is how things play out: First, after you drink, alcohol enters your baby's blood circulation through the placenta, increasing his blood-alcohol concentration to mirror your own. From this entry point, alcohol reaches all the cells in his body, including his brain. Because your baby's liver doesn't yet function like an adult's, alcohol stays in his system longer than it does in yours. This prolonged exposure disrupts development. Indeed, alcohol is defined as a **teratogen**—a substance that is known to interfere with normal fetal development and cause structural or functional abnormalities. (The word comes from the Greek *téras*, meaning "monster," and *gen*, "to produce"—literally, "monster-producer." Yikes.)

And in extreme cases of heavy drinking (more than seven standard drinks per week or more than four or five drinks per occasion—within two hours—on at least two occasions), a baby can develop what is called Fetal Alcohol Syndrome (FAS). This condition causes permanent changes to the child's brain and body because the fetus develops in a toxic environment. Symptoms can include distinctive facial features, growth restriction, and lifelong cognitive and behavioral difficulties.

When pregnant mice were given alcohol levels that mimicked a glass of wine a day in humans, their pups grew up with measurable changes in behavior. They had more trouble focusing, made more mistakes on attention tasks, and reacted more impulsively than pups from moms that weren't given any alcohol. Other experiments found that baby rats exposed to moderate alcohol before birth seemed outwardly normal at first—same size, same litter numbers—but as they matured, their social behavior shifted. They played more aggressively, wrestled more, and were less curious about new peers compared to alcohol-free controls. Reviews that look at dozens of these animal studies show the same pattern: moderate prenatal alcohol exposure can leave invisible fingerprints on the brain—poorer memory, weaker motor coordination, unusual social interactions, and a heightened stress response that can last into adulthood. In other words, even if the baby looks healthy at birth, their wiring may be subtly altered in ways that show up only years later.

This is why public health agencies, including the World Health Organization and the Centers for Disease Control (CDC), recommend complete abstinence during pregnancy. You get it: avoid alcohol.

During breastfeeding, however, it's a different story. It's not like pregnancy, when your baby is directly connected to your bloodstream and exposed to whatever is circulating there at all times. If you are moderately drinking, like one glass, as long as you wait two to three hours before breastfeeding, the amount in breast milk becomes negligible. If you drink more than that, it will take much longer to leave your system and to not show up in your breast milk. Okay—on to our next substance.

Coffee and tea

I'm a coffee addict. Every few months I try to quit because even one morning cup can mess with my sleep, but I never quite manage. I just love it too much. During pregnancy, though, reducing my coffee intake became a real goal. It was the first time in my life I actually cut back.

In the first trimester, high caffeine intake has been linked to a greater risk of early miscarriage, even before implantation. Because of my past miscarriage, I was especially diligent about this and it was very easy to skip my morning cappuccino. In the later trimesters, I kept my intake low as well (although it wasn't zero). While moderate caffeine is generally considered safe in pregnancy, there are a few biological mechanisms worth knowing about that explain why too much can be a problem.

When you're not pregnant, half the caffeine from your morning latte is gone from your blood within three to five hours. By the third trimester of pregnancy, things have drastically changed: it takes closer to *ten hours*! We become worse at clearing caffeine as pregnancy progresses—meaning that same cup of coffee will keep you wired for longer in your third trimester than in your second. This slowdown likely happens because your body shifts caffeine clearance down the priority list, allowing the liver to focus on more essential functions. (This also means that you can drink less coffee than before and will feel the effects for longer. If you're dealing with insomnia, know that your usual cup is affecting you much more than before.)

But, once again, caffeine in your bloodstream doesn't stop with you. Just like with alcohol, caffeine crosses the placenta freely, and your baby's blood levels of caffeine mirror yours. In other words, you're sharing your espresso shot. The problem is that your baby's liver isn't yet equipped to break down caffeine at all. So while you eventually clear it, in his circulation it lingers much, much longer.

Today, around 70 percent of pregnant moms consume caffeine during their pregnancy. And their babies seem to respond to it: studies find that after drinking coffee, a baby in the womb is awake for longer and his heart rate increases.

There are a few biological reasons to suspect caffeine could be harmful. It narrows blood vessels, including those in the placenta, reducing oxygen and nutrient delivery. It also blocks adenosine, a molecule critical for fetal growth and brain wiring. In animal experiments, prenatal caffeine exposure has been shown to produce smaller pups, alter the pups' heart development, and delay brain maturation.

In humans, we don't have direct clinical trial data on the long-term impact of caffeine during pregnancy. No one is running studies where one group of women is asked to drink lots of coffee while another abstains completely. What we do have are observational studies. And these show that higher caffeine intake in pregnancy is associated with smaller babies. One large UK study even found a higher risk of low birth weight at moderate intakes (equivalent to two shots of espresso a day), although, of course, we can't fully rule out confounding factors. All that said, research finds very few long-term effects of caffeine on human babies: some association studies report subtle alterations of the brains of kids at ten years old who were born to moms who drank a lot of caffeine while pregnant. But the research certainly doesn't paint caffeine as catastrophic. Overall, there are no significant links between caffeine during pregnancy and the long-term neurodevelopment of children.

This is why public health agencies stop short of calling for zero caffeine, instead advising limits. The European Food Safety Authority and the American College of Obstetricians and Gynecologists, for example, both recommend keeping caffeine under 200mg per day (roughly the amount in one large 350ml cup of brewed coffee, or three shots of espresso, or four cups of black tea).

Put together, the safest, simplest rule is: keep it to one cup a day, and if it's all the same to you, switch to decaf. Also remember to count hidden sources (tea, cola, energy drinks, chocolate). Caffeine is not alcohol—it's not a neurotoxin—but it can still have an effect on you and your baby.

I actually tracked how many days I went without coffee during my pregnancy. It went something like this: first trimester—perfect score. Second trimester—I drank coffee on 20 percent of the days. Third trimester: I drank coffee on 40 percent of the days. (PS: The first place I rushed to after going home with my newborn from the hospital? My favorite coffee shop.)

During breastfeeding, things get easier: **only 1 percent of the caffeine you drink makes its way into your breast milk.** Health authorities still suggest keeping caffeine below 300mg a day during breastfeeding (roughly five shots of espresso). So you don't need to worry about one cup, although if your baby seems very jittery, restless or wakes easily, you can try cutting down on caffeine to see if that could be the cause.

Broccoli and stretch marks

If you've been moving through this book and noticed I haven't said much about the produce section of the supermarket, that was not a mistake. It's because the structural molecules that build your baby's body aren't in broccoli or apples: they are mostly proteins (amino acids, which become muscle, skin, and organs) found in foods like meat, eggs, dairy, beans and pulses; and fats (lipids, which form cell membranes and the growing brain) found in foods like fish, nuts, seeds, avocado, and olive oil.

Fruit and vegetables, by contrast, are low in protein and fat, so they don't directly provide those building blocks. They do bring carbohydrates, which turn to glucose—and provide energy. But what they excel at above all are micronutrients: vitamins (like folate, vitamin C, and vitamin K), minerals (like potassium and magnesium), plus a whole array of phytonutrients (like carotenoids, flavonoids, and polyphenols). These are the tools that make construction in your womb possible: they help enzymes work, protect cells from damage, and ensure proper development.

If you're curious, many of the beneficial compounds in produce are also the reason that the fruit and veg are colorful: carotenoids (orange and yellow), anthocyanins (red, blue, purple), and chlorophylls (deep green). Dark leafy greens such as kale and spinach are loaded with folate, vitamin K, and lutein, which supports eye and brain development. Orange vegetables like carrots and sweet potatoes are dense in beta-carotene, a precursor to vitamin A that is critical for your baby's immunity. Red, purple, and blue foods like berries and eggplant contain anthocyanins and flavonoids, potent antioxidants that help lower inflammation. **A good rule of thumb: the deeper and more vibrant the color of a plant, the richer it tends to be in vitamins, antioxidants, polyphenols, and other phytonutrients. So, when you're filling your plate, let color be your guide.** If it's dark, if it's vibrant, if it stains your cutting board—go for it.

Here's an example: When I was five months pregnant and on a plane, I was served a not-very-good quinoa galette, but there were beautiful peppers around it. Red, green, yellow peppers. Now, guess what: I hate peppers. I just don't like them. I don't get them. Well, I ate them anyway. (A mother's sacrifice.) Why? Because those vibrant colors signal the presence of vitamins and phytonutrients like carotenoids and flavonoids: powerful antioxidants that I knew would protect cells and support my baby's development.

While a standard prenatal supplement will provide many of these micronutrients, it's always a better idea to get them from food. First, we often absorb them more efficiently when they come packaged in whole foods. Nutrients in real foods arrive alongside complementary compounds that help the body use them well.

What about fiber? Fiber in fruits and vegetables has plenty of benefits for you, like keeping your glucose levels steady, feeding your gut microbes (more on this in the next section), and helping digestion. But none of it reaches your baby directly. By design, fiber stays in your intestines and never crosses into the bloodstream, so it can't end up in your baby's circulation. And that's fine—your baby doesn't need fiber in the womb. What does matter is that when you eat fiber, your gut bacteria thrive and become more diverse. A healthy microbiome produces compounds that lower inflammation in your body, creating a better environment for your baby's growth and development. That's a win for you and your baby.

There's one last bit of magic here: as I explained in Chapter 1, your baby can "taste" foods in the womb. Flavors from your diet pass into the amniotic fluid and shape early food preferences, easing your child's path toward accepting a mouthful of spinach later on. A study even showed newborns responded more positively to the smell of carrot or kale if their mothers consumed those during pregnancy.

Oh, and **a quick note on fruit and vegetables and stretch marks**: unfortunately no topical applications such as shea butter or olive oil actually seem to prevent them. What can help is massaging your skin. But to help your skin stretch from within, your body needs amino acids (from protein) to build new collagen, and vitamin C. An essential cofactor for collagen synthesis, vitamin C helps enzymes link collagen fibers together, making them stronger and more elastic. Without enough of it, collagen can't form properly. That's why oranges, strawberries, kiwis, and, yes—even peppers (sigh)—are excellent for your skin and supportive of it stretching during pregnancy. However, even with the best care and nutrition, some women will still get stretch marks, as genetics, ethnicity, and skin type all play a major role in whether they appear. (By the way, peppers and I have reconciled thanks to a tahini dressing you'll find in The Baby Salad recipe on page 302.)

Fermented foods and probiotics

Very early research suggests that a more diverse microbiome during pregnancy can help your baby's immune system develop better. That's because the microbes in your gut don't just sit there. They send out tiny chemical signals that can reach your baby through the placenta. A wider variety of microbes means a wider variety of signals, which may help your baby's immune system learn and get stronger before birth.

For example, a review of 19 randomized trials found that when mothers took probiotic supplements during late pregnancy and breastfeeding, their children had about a 22 percent lower risk of developing eczema in early life. We don't yet fully understand the mechanism, but it seems that when a mom adds "good bacteria," it helps to prime her baby's immune system to be less overreactive (just like we saw with omega-3s and inflammation).

Fermented foods may add more benefits. In animal models, fermented maternal diets have produced dramatic shifts: piglets and mouse pups born to mothers fed a fermented "super-diet" developed guts rich in *Lactobacillus* (a type of "good" bacteria), with better intestinal function and reduced inflammation. It's early days for this research but already the takeaway is exciting: by shaping your own microbiome with supplements and fermented foods, you may be helping to program your baby's immune defenses for years to come.

Fermented foods are generally safe in pregnancy, but there is a key point to keep in mind: always pick pasteurized versions to avoid harmful microbes. The good news is that pasteurization doesn't necessarily wipe out the beneficial bacteria, because most yogurts and kefirs are pasteurized first, then live cultures are added back in.

Some foods to have once in a while, if you feel like it, are:

- → **Yogurt:** Pick plain, unsweetened versions with live cultures (all the traditional yogurt brands have these in them). This is an easy base to make My Absolute Favorite Snack (see page 304).
- → **Kefir:** A drinkable, tangier cousin of yogurt, loaded with diverse probiotics.
- → **Sauerkraut and kimchi:** Fermented cabbage dishes that deliver crunch and a probiotic punch. (Commercial kimchi sold in the refrigerated section is generally considered safe, because it's produced under controlled conditions, but check with your doctor.)
- → **Natto:** A Japanese staple made from fermented soy beans that is rich in both probiotics and vitamin K2. An acquired taste, but powerful for gut health.

Plastic

When I was pregnant, I suddenly started looking at the plastics in my life with suspicion. The Invisalign trays I had worn every night? I put them away. Heating leftovers in plastic containers? Stopped. Plastic water bottles? Bye-bye. I switched to glass and stainless steel instead. These changes were rooted in an important piece of information: plastics aren't neutral. They shed chemicals like bisphenols and phthalates that slip into our food and our bodies. They even break down into microplastics, which scientists have now found **lodged in human placentas in 80–100 percent of samples studied**. And microplastics are also found in breast milk in 76 percent of samples. What's the impact? It's unclear for now, but it can't be good: we know, for example, that microplastics damage cells and disrupt biological processes. That means our baby's first home is not as untouched as we'd like to imagine.

Here's what you can actively do to try to minimize the amount of chemicals and microplastics from entering your system:

→ Use glass, ceramic, or stainless steel for food and drink, especially for hot items.
→ Never microwave plastic containers or bottles: heat accelerates chemical leaching.
→ Choose fresh or frozen foods over canned goods (which are often lined with bisphenols).
→ Swap plastic wrap with beeswax or reusable covers.

→ Pick phthalate-free personal care products (look for labels or simpler ingredient lists).
→ Limit your handling of receipts, which are coated with BPA, or wash your hands after contact. (I know it makes me look crazy, but I try to grab receipts between my nails instead of with my fingers . . .)

Giving birth

This may go without saying: I'm not a midwife. What follows is grounded in the latest scientific research, but your care team's advice should always be what guides your decisions.

First things first, we cannot know in advance how our labor will unfold. All we can do is prepare, make choices that align with our hopes, and then adapt. There is no hierarchy of birth (vaginal birth isn't "better" than a C-section)—there is only the truth that you brought a new human into the world. No matter how your baby arrives, he's here, and you did something extraordinary.

Now, let's look at the science. One of the clearest findings in childbirth research is this: continuous support during labor—from a midwife, a doula (a trained birth companion), a partner, or even a trusted friend—improves outcomes. By contrast, standard medical care often means being left alone for stretches of time, with staff coming in only periodically to check on progress.

The difference is remarkable. When a midwife or a doula is present, offering touch, massage, eye contact, reassurance, the perceived pain of labor drops. **The need for pain medication or an epidural falls from 83 percent to 72 percent.** Labor itself becomes shorter by an average of *two hours*. And, most strikingly, the rate of emergency C-sections is cut by up to half.

That's powerful, because C-sections are often seen as purely mechanical events—something that happens only if the baby is stuck or complications arise. But the data shows otherwise.

When a mother feels supported, her hormones flow, her body labors more efficiently, and the chance of surgical intervention is dramatically reduced. (Of course, sometimes a C-section is absolutely necessary, with or without a doula. But support during labor can shift the odds in your favor in profound ways.)

How do we know this? Well, because of what we know about a very special molecule called **oxytocin**. The great orchestrator of your labor, oxytocin is released by your brain in the weeks leading up to your baby's birth, and in a much higher dose on the day your labor actually starts. Oxytocin binds to receptors on your uterus, causing contractions and also stimulating the release of prostaglandins (the omega-6–derived molecules that we saw in Chapter 4 that soften your cervix). For labor to be efficient and progress naturally, oxytocin is vital. But there is a twist: it's a very shy hormone.

Here's a thought experiment: oxytocin is the same hormone that gets released when we have sex. What do you need for sex? Intimacy, warmth, dim lights, a sense of safety. You don't want to be hungry or thirsty. You don't want bright lights, interruptions, a ticking clock, or being told whether you are doing it right or not. You (probably?) don't want strangers staring at you. Well, for oxytocin to flow during labor, you need exactly the same conditions. This same hormone that drives orgasm also drives contractions. If the setting helps oxytocin during sex, it will help oxytocin during labor. That's why a calm environment, dark room, loving touch, and **continuous support from a doula, friend, or partner, aren't "extras": they are biological enablers of labor**. And it's why the studies find that this kind of support improves labor outcomes. You can easily understand how the traditional hospital room with bright lights, people coming in and out, or loud voices, can stall natural labor; and why it's more likely to lead to interventions or to the use of synthetic oxytocin (pitocin).

This is why it's so important to build your support, and create a **birth plan**: write it out, print it, and share it with your medical team ahead of time. Your plan can include anything that helps you feel safe and comfortable: low lights, hushed voices, no updates on how many hours have passed, and reminders not to mention dilation numbers if you'd rather not know. You can bring familiar objects, fairy lights, your favorite playlist, or your favorite snacks. Meeting the people who will be in the room ahead of time also makes a difference—recognizing a face or two can feel grounding when things get intense. I even bought blackout shades for the car windows so I wouldn't feel observed during the drive from home to the hospital. It's your birth, and the details are up to you. If it helps, I've put my own birth plan on my website so you can see exactly what I asked for. Find it at this link glucosegoddess.com/pages/birth-plan (or by scanning the QR code below). (I was at a physiological-forward hospital—a hospital that encourages intervention-free births—so didn't need to add things like no episiotomy, and so on, but those are things you can list as well.)

My birth plan

Should you eat dates to speed up labor?

You might ask why anyone would wonder such a thing, but this is one of the most common questions I get. In some cultures, notably in the Middle East, midwives have long recommended that women eat dates toward the end of pregnancy to help speed up labor when it comes. A while back, some scientists picked up on this and decided to test if there was something measurable behind the tradition.

And . . . the results were mixed. Some studies showed that eating six dates per day during later pregnancy can reduce labor time. But they were small studies and had some methodology flaws. Most importantly of all, though, the studies did not look at the downsides of what dates do to your glucose levels. Indeed, any potential benefit of speeding up labor is strongly countered by the immense amount of sugar contained in dates.

In six dried dates, you will find 27g of sugar. This is more than the daily 25g WHO recommendation of maximum amount of sugar intake per day. On the following page you'll find a graph showing the glucose spike a friend of mine experienced after eating six dried dates when she was seven months pregnant. As you can clearly see: massive spike. (Incredibly, dried dates are actually recommended as a "healthy" snack for people with type 2 diabetes, who must keep their glucose levels steady as a matter of urgency. Shocking, I know.)

As we saw in Chapter 1, the sugar in dates does not get a free pass just because it comes from fruit. It's still sugar.

Consuming six dried dates per day, as some people might recommend, is a one-way ticket to a giant glucose roller coaster, with massive daily glucose spikes. Those six dates also mean your baby will receive a large influx of sugar—and he will need to release insulin to manage it . . . and so on.

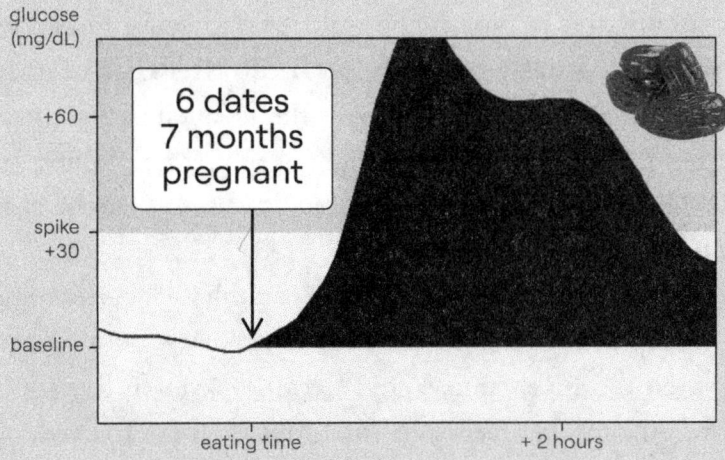

Dates may improve labour timing. But at what cost to our glucose levels?

If you really want to eat dates, reduce the spike by eating them only after a meal, and putting "clothing" on them (see page 84) and never eat them on an empty stomach. The fact remains: dried dates—like any dried fruit—are a source of sugar.

And, as you've just learned, there are other things proven to make labor faster and less painful—that *don't* come with a glucose spike!

Banishing the fear factor

Now, while there may be lots of things that trigger stress feelings during labor that you can't control, the one thing you can control is the pervasive societally induced fear around childbirth. I know how common this is, because I was full of it myself. Before I was even pregnant, I was wholeheartedly **TER-RI-FIED** of giving birth. I imagined chaos—rushing to the hospital, screaming in pain from the very first contraction, hooked up to machines, surrounded by interventions. In my mind, it was going to be absolutely horrible.

I wanted to unpack all this fear so I could have a better mindset as I prepared, and stack the odds in my favor for a peaceful birth when the time came. Why? Because oxytocin flows most easily when a mother feels safe, supported, and unobserved, and is inhibited by stress hormones like adrenaline, which pump through our body when we feel afraid.

I didn't want to feel afraid. I don't want you to feel afraid. So here's what I learned.

Movies have really messed with our heads. They almost always show birth as a frantic, bloody crisis, with lots of shouting. This image is so pervasive that, for many of us, it's the only one we carry. But real birth looks very different. Contractions usually build gradually, and it often takes many hours (or days) before you even leave for your birthplace. In most cases, there's no need for a dramatic rush through traffic in an ambulance with sirens blaring.

The stories we tell ourselves matter, and if all we know are scenes of panic, it's no wonder we go into birth with fear. I had to consciously replace those images with new ones. I began watching videos of women giving birth naturally, calmly and with confidence. It changed everything for me. If you're preparing for your own labor, I can't recommend this enough: search for "positive birth stories" and flood your mind with examples of what birth can look like when women are supported and safe.

Of course, birth used to kill mothers. That's the most common argument for medicalizing it. It's true that childbirth can be dangerous. Before antibiotics, sterile tools, or blood transfusions, many women died from infection, hemorrhage, or obstructed labor. In the 1800s, maternal mortality in Europe and North America was estimated to be as high as one in 100 births. Today, in high-income countries, that number is closer to one in 8,300 vaginal births.

Modern medicine is essential when emergencies happen, and thank goodness we have it. But the pendulum has swung too far: instead of focusing on the small minority of births that truly require intervention, we've built a system that treats all births as needing medical support. In reality, around 98 percent of births unfold without life-threatening complications. Birth should be supported as a normal physiological event—with medical care available if needed, but not imposed by default. The story that a doctor is needed for a birth isn't neutral; it's cultural conditioning. And culture shapes outcomes. In the Netherlands, about half of women give birth without an epidural. In France, it's closer to 10 percent. Do Dutch women feel less pain? No. Their society gives them more confidence, more reassurance that giving birth is natural and that they can do it.

And they're right. Your body is built for this. The uterus is the strongest muscle in the human body by weight. Contractions aren't random pain—they are the most powerful and purposeful movements your body will ever make. Reframing pain as progress changes the experience. Let's unpack what happens, step by step.

The first stage of labor

Let's talk about your cervix. The first stage of labor is when the cervix, the passage between your uterus and your vagina, softens, thins, then opens to 10cm in diameter. This first stage of labor is broken down into two phases: the *latent phase*, when contractions are still irregular, relatively mild, and the cervix is slowly softening and beginning to dilate (up to about 3–4cm). The *active phase* follows, when contractions become stronger, longer, and more regular, and the cervix dilates more rapidly.

It's a process. Under the influence of oxytocin, your uterus contracts, and as I say, this pressure first leads to the effacement, or thinning, of your cervix.

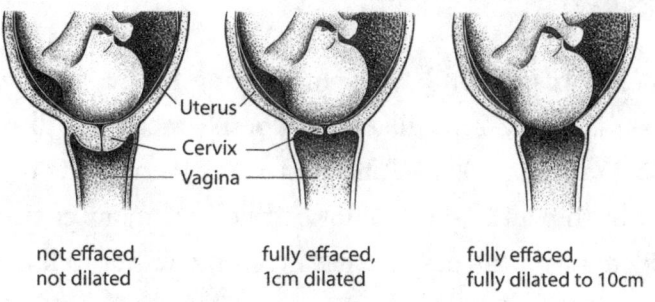

not effaced, not dilatedfully effaced, 1cm dilatedfully effaced, fully dilated to 10cm

Your cervix does two things: first it effaces, then it dilates.

Then, your cervix will *dilate*, meaning it will open. This is a term most of us are familiar with ("You are x centimeters dilated"). But one thing to note here: cervical dilation does not progress in a straight line—the first 2–4cm often take far longer than the last 6cm, as you see in the graph on page 234. So, **when someone says "You're only two centimeters dilated," remember: much of the hardest, longest** groundwork of cervical *effacing* is already done, because the first centimeters of dilation are the longest. Being 2cm dilated is already quite advanced into the process.

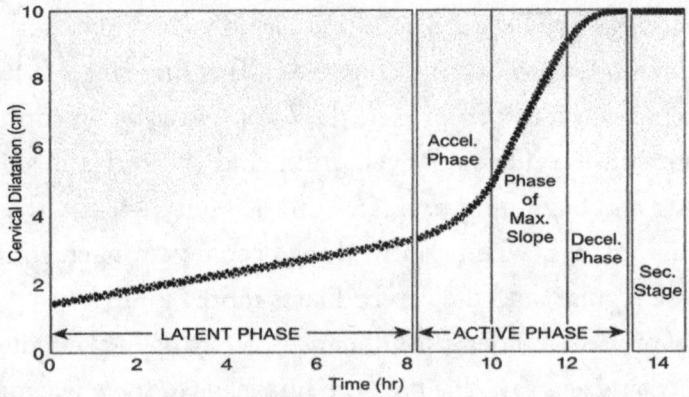

The first phase of labor (cervical effacement and dilation) is broken down into latent and active phases. The active phase is generally when you'll be admitted to the hospital (if you are having a hospital birth).

In other words, if you have been laboring for five hours and are told you are only 2cm dilated, it doesn't mean it will take you 20 hours to get to 10cm. You could get to 10cm in the next hour. (In my birth plan I asked to not be told how many centimeters I was dilated; you can ask for that if you prefer not to know.)

Anyway, getting from a closed cervix to one that is fully effaced and dilated (aka having gone through the entire first stage of labor) can take anything from six hours to three days. The contractions felt to me like stronger and stronger period pains, building gradually.

What helps: Ignore the contractions as long as possible until they really start to build. Keep life normal. Walk, eat, cuddle, nap, watch TV. Don't watch the clock. Once the contractions get intense, go into your "bubble" (wherever you feel safe, in your bedroom with dim lights on a birth ball, for example), and reach for pain management tools—birth combs, counter-pressure, hip squeezes, acupressure. Try breathing techniques, keeping your face relaxed to diffuse tension ("loose jaw, soft forehead"); vocalize low sounds; change positions every 30 minutes. Hydration (water, coconut water) and snacks are good (trail mix was my best friend!).

Mindset matters: Remember, oxytocin is shy—dim lights, warmth, no observers.

* TOP TIPS *

* **Bath:** Here is a tip I got from my midwife that turned out to be very helpful (but there is no strong published evidence on the topic): going into a bath when you're in the latent phase may slow down labor, which is why it's generally reserved for active labor. In fact, she told me that this is a way of telling what stage you're in: if contractions slow down when you're in hot water, you're still early. If they keep going, you're shifting into active labor. This turned out to perfectly match my experience.

* **Position matters:** Lying on your back is the hardest way to labor, it narrows the pelvis and makes contractions feel sharper. It also slows things down and increases the likelihood of needing instruments. Squatting, standing, kneeling, swaying, even sitting on the toilet—all of these positions widen the pelvis and work with gravity. As much as you can, continue to move, even once you are at the hospital. Science shows that lying down on

your back makes this first stage of labor, on average, **1 hour and 22 minutes longer** than it is for women who are upright, walking and moving. Women who move during labor are also less likely to have a C-section and an epidural (being on your back hurts much more than staying on the move during the contractions).

The second and third stages of labor

The second stage of labor begins once your cervix is fully effaced and fully dilated to 10cm. This is the point when your baby can begin to move down into your pelvis and birth canal. With each contraction, your uterus pushes the baby lower. At first, this may feel like pressure deep in your pelvis or rectum. As your baby descends, contractions tend to shift from being primarily painful to being more about the urge to push. For me, the sign of change came as the tail end of each contraction turned into the pushing reflex, and then gradually more and more of the duration of the contraction was about pushing, until it was just that. Pushing.

Your role: Even though we often say "pushing," much of this stage is actually your body doing the work reflexively. Your job is to follow the urge, stay as relaxed as possible between contractions, and conserve energy.

What helps: Upright positions (squatting, kneeling, on hands-and-knees), which as I mentioned in the first labor stage, widen the pelvis and use gravity. Vocalizing in low tones like a moan, breathing in rhythm, and having continuous support make a difference. Trust the reflex. Vocalize before the peak of the contraction. Partners can support with grounding phrases ("One minute, we'll do it together").

The second stage of labor ends when your baby is born. And ideally, he is placed right on to your chest for skin-to-skin contact. Skin-to-skin helps regulate your baby's breathing, temperature and heart rate, stabilizes blood glucose, and even seeds their microbiome with your bacteria. This first hour together is often called the golden hour, and it has profound physiological benefits. Early skin-to-skin promotes the release of oxytocin in both mother and baby, which strengthens bonding, calms stress responses, and primes your baby's brain for neurodevelopment. It also helps clear fluid from the lungs, encourages the newborn's instinctive crawl to the breast, and sets the stage for successful breastfeeding.

After that comes the third stage of labor: delivering the placenta. Your uterus continues to contract, this time to help the placenta separate and expel. These contractions are vital not just for completing the birth but for closing off blood vessels and preventing haemorrhage.

Medical interventions

Medical interventions during birth are sometimes necessary and life-saving. There is no question about that. Here are a few science-backed tips for them. First, if you are **being induced**, one option worth discussing with your care team is, rather than be injected with **synthetic oxytocin from the get-go**, to insert a **prostaglandin tampon**. Prostaglandins help soften the cervix and can sometimes initiate contractions. For many people, this creates a more gradual start to labor compared with being induced with synthetic oxytocin. Experiences vary, though, and the right approach will depend on your individual situation.

In the case of a **C-section**, your baby will not pass through the birth canal. Normally, during vaginal birth, a baby is exposed to the mother's microbiome—tiny communities of bacteria that help "seed" the baby's gut and immune system. This early exposure is thought to be helpful for the development of your baby's microbiome. One approach that some parents consider after a C-section is called **"vaginal seeding"**—using a swab from the mother's vagina to gently wipe the baby's mouth, face, or body to transfer some of those microbes. There is not enough research on this yet to confirm its efficacy and safety, but if this is something you're interested in, talk with your care team in advance. In some hospitals, you can have vaginal seeding under medical supervision.

My birth story

I want to tell you my story because as I was pregnant I craved hearing other people's stories, especially the unfiltered raw truth. There are as many birth stories as there are births, but listening to them helped me prepare for my own. So here we go!

It took me a long time to find the right care team. I met with four different hospitals before choosing the one where it finally felt right. Each place subscribed to its own philosophy, and carried its own energy. Each had a different outlook on interventions, and different guidelines for water births (which is what I was hoping for). Only a few accepted doulas in addition to partners in the room—and I realized how much this mattered to me. I had a no-intervention natural birth plan, but didn't want to do a home birth, so I wanted to find a place that corresponded to my wishes as much as possible.

Finding a doula I trusted made a huge difference too. I started seeing her for monthly sessions when I was in my first trimester of pregnancy. Knowing she would be there on the day of the birth helped me to feel less fearful about the process as well. My husband prepared too—he read a book called *The Birth Partner*, and came to the hospital with me equipped with phrases, counter-pressure moves, and confidence. We also wrote a detailed birth plan to help everyone understand what mattered to us when the time came.

Labor began on a Sunday morning, like period pains that got stronger, little by little. From 9 a.m. until late noon, we mostly went about our day as usual: that was part of our plan to not get exhausted too early. We cuddled, ate lunch, walked around, timed contractions. By early afternoon when the pains hit a new level, I needed to sit down during the contractions. That's when I asked my husband to hold a hot-water bottle on my lower back. I remember thinking: "This hurts, but I'm happy. I'm handling it."

We set up a little "birth bubble" in my bedroom—blinds drawn, cozy and private. During contractions, I leaned into my husband's arms and he counted to 20 with me. The whole time he was in the room with me, chatting, present, by my side. Sometimes I squeezed a birth comb into my palm (it helped to focus on that sharp pressure instead of the contraction pain). We laughed a lot. It was manageable but the idea of leaving the room or standing up felt a bit much. (Fun fact: I even decided to pee in a vase in my room instead of getting up to go to the bathroom, because walking down the corridor felt way too hard an undertaking.)

By midafternoon, the contractions were getting more intense. I was in my bubble, just focusing on each as they came, and resting in between. I had to moan through them—long, low sounds that seemed to carry me through the pain. The clock was telling us that the contractions were three minutes apart, lasting one minute, and this had been going on for over an hour. Based on our natural birth plan, this was our cue to go to the hospital. I didn't really want to get in the car because I was very much in my bubble, but it was clear we should go.

Getting into the car felt like a milestone. Contractions slowed down a little on the journey, giving me precious moments of rest between the waves (I was less relaxed, my oxytocin was probably lowering as I left my bubble). When they did hit, I held on to the car door handle and groaned my way through each one.

At the maternity ward, a male midwife asked me to pee in a cup to check something, which was *supremely* annoying at that point. He wasn't particularly kind. He even wanted to draw blood—I flat out refused. This felt completely insane considering the level of pain I was in. He checked me and told me I was 5cm dilated, although I hadn't wanted to know the number. Just then, my doula Elsa arrived, smiling and full of encouragement. I was glad to see her. She knew our plan, I felt reassured having her there with me.

From here, things got serious. I spent another three hours in the dimly lit birth room, alternating between sitting on the birth ball, standing and leaning against the bed, or sitting in the water bath, gripping Elsa's hand during every single contraction. As soon as each contraction started, I shouted her name: "ELSA!" I needed to hold on to her to survive it. Visualizations helped too—I pictured my favorite vacation spot and told myself, "Three long ommmmmms and it will be over." At this point, my husband might as well not have been there, it would have made no difference. His one job was to rest the hot water bottle on my back when I leaned against the bed and even that I felt like he was doing wrong. So I kept screaming at him (I'm sorry, honey).

The pain was overwhelming, deep in my bones, like an unoiled machine creaking my body open. I moved my legs constantly by total reflex, trying to find space in my pelvis. What made it exhausting was not getting any breaks—the contractions were now relentless. I kept thinking, when is this going to stop?

Elsa reassured me: "Your baby will be born soon." At that point, I began to feel the urge to push at the end of contractions. Slowly, the sensation grew stronger. My waters finally broke. It felt like a balloon bursting inside me. The pain was now sharper, much sharper than I expected, almost unbearable. I told Elsa I couldn't take it anymore and even asked for the epidural—using our code word. She told me it was too late, and reminded me gently that I was in a negative thought pattern and encouraged me to say "YES" to the next contractions instead of resisting. It helped, but it was still the hardest thing I've ever endured. It hurt like hell.

Then came the shift: the irresistible urge to push. The power of it was insane. It was no longer about me choosing; my body was doing it on its own.

I felt his head moving down, the pressure like a giant watermelon. (A friend had said giving birth feels like the biggest poop of your life. I concur.) Two more contractions, pushing with every ounce of strength I had left, while kneeling. A burning stretch, then my son was born! I was a total wreck and euphoric at the same time.

Oh, and I was wearing my glucose sensor the whole time:

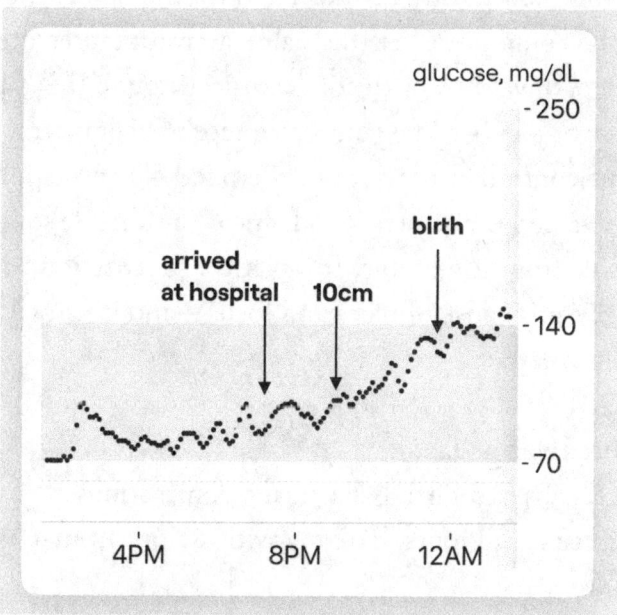

What you'll notice is the rise in my glucose levels as birth progressed, even though I didn't eat anything between 6 p.m. and midnight. This was as a result of cortisol rising and my body releasing glucose into my bloodstream to help my uterus have enough fuel to do its job.

Pain management and labor kit

Labor hurts. There's no two ways around it. We all perceive pain differently, so it's impossible to know how it will feel *for you*. Personally, even with a doula, a supportive medical team, and lots of knowledge, it hurt like hell for me (I used no drugs, and if I were to rate it, I would say it was 15-out-of-ten pain). However, your body has a built-in mechanism to support you through it: it releases endorphins—natural opioids that rise in response to contractions. With movement, touch, and calm, endorphins can help pain become a bit more bearable.

One of the things I did use was a **birth comb**. This is a simple tool you hold tightly in your hand during contractions. The teeth of the comb press into the palm, activating pressure points and nerve pathways. A birth comb works through the "gate control theory of pain": when your brain receives competing signals (sharp but controlled pressure in the hand + contraction pain), the non-harmful pressure helps "distract" or override some of the pain signals from the uterus. In practice, squeezing a comb can give a surprising sense of relief and focus—and it's small enough to take anywhere.

What I used during labor:
→ Birth combs and birth balls during contractions
→ Positions: on all fours, hanging with a cloth from a doorframe
→ Hip squeezes from my partner, acupressure points
→ Large jugs of coconut water for hydration

→ During contractions, I inhaled thinking about bringing oxygen to the baby, and I exhaled imagining I was a balloon deflating
→ Deep moans—simply breathing during contractions was often not enough to help my body relax and soften, so I tried deep moans instead
→ When feeling labor pains in the back, the "lift and pelvic tuck" technique was useful to help my baby engage in the pelvis and cervix instead of pressing against my back

My labor kit:
→ ChapStick
→ Eye mask
→ Small lights to use at home and at the hospital
→ Birth combs and birth balls
→ Water mister
→ Electrolytes to put in water
→ Large 2-liter water jug with a straw to be able to drink in any position

Breastfeeding and formula

This book is about pregnancy nutrition—but the truth is, the story doesn't end when your baby is born. As we've seen, the first 1,000 days are when the most critical programming for long-term health takes place. The food a baby receives in the first two years also influences his health for life. And for the first six months, breast milk or formula is basically the whole menu. Before we look at how to pick formula, first, let's cover a few reasons why breast milk is different.

First, breast milk is **alive with information**. As we saw in Chapter 1, it carries tiny epigenetic messengers called RNAs. These microscopic regulators survive digestion, enter your baby's bloodstream, and attach to DNA, fine-tuning how genes are expressed after every feed. Some of the most abundant RNAs in breast milk are linked to immune development and brain function. This may help explain why breastfed babies often show stronger immune defenses, sharper metabolic regulation, and lower risks of obesity, asthma, blood pressure, and certain infections later in life. Your breast milk also contains healthy bacteria that help seed your baby's microbiome. In other words, every feed is not just nutrition—it's programming for lifelong health.

Second, your breast milk **adapts in real time**. As your baby grows, the balance of fat, protein, hormones, and RNAs changes. And, if your baby is fighting an infection, your milk immediately shifts—upping its immune cells, antibodies, and bioactive factors. It's a personalized, dynamic system that responds to your child's needs day by day. No two breast milks are the same: yours is unique to you and your baby.

It also contains everything your baby needs. These remarkable properties are thought to be why longer durations of breastfeeding are linked to lower rates of childhood obesity, diabetes, and allergies, and even help nurture healthier gut bacteria that persist after weaning. One 2025 study showed that babies breastfed for at least six months were up to 27 percent less likely to have developmental delays later on. Breast milk doesn't just nourish—it gives babies a measurable edge in brain development. Research shows that babies breastfed for at least three months have **20–30 percent more white matter** in their brains, meaning the wiring in their brain was more developed. And even after accounting for maternal intelligence, children who were breastfed outperformed those who were formula-fed in the long term—scoring 2–3 points higher on cognitive tests well into their *teenage years*.

If you are breastfeeding, do remember to keep your protein, choline, and DHA levels up. This is extremely important. These key nutrients continue being transferred to your child's developing body and brain, and the amount transferred is in direct correlation with how much you ingest.

In fact, breastfeeding demands *more* of these nutrients than during the third trimester of pregnancy (shocking, I know!), because your baby is now bigger and relies entirely on your breast milk for growth. So keep up your choline (550mg+ daily up from 450mg+), protein (1.9g per kilogram of bodyweight per day, up from 1.52g), and DHA (300mg+ daily) intake. Refer to the table on page 256 for exact amounts.

In terms of overall calories, it's the same story: you need more than during pregnancy because making milk is very demanding (milk production uses about 500kcal/day per baby in the first six months. If you have twins, it's about 1,000kcal/day). If you eat too little food, you may feel weaker. I noticed this myself: About a month postpartum, I could see a strong correlation between how much I ate and my mental state. If I didn't eat a ton of food, I would feel depleted and very low.

That being said, not everyone can or wants to breastfeed. If your baby is formula fed, the great news is that formula is highly regulated: the basics of protein, carbohydrate, fat, vitamins, and minerals are standardized across all approved brands. So your baby will always get the essential building blocks he needs.

But pay special attention to the ingredient list of your formula, and check for two often overlooked molecules you've learned about in this book: DHA and choline.

Every day, a breastfeeding mother passes 50–80mg of DHA to her baby. Recognizing its importance, Europe made DHA mandatory in infant formulas in 2021. In the US, though, it's still only "recommended," not required (as of 2025). So wherever you are, check the label and make sure it's there.

Choline is just as vital. In the first six months of life, a baby needs around 125mg per day, and 150mg per day from seven to twelve months. This is the amount that gets passed through breast milk. Yet formula choline levels vary widely, and unlike DHA, they aren't consistently regulated. Some formulas still fall short, or contain no choline at all, so don't assume it's covered—confirm the amount before you buy.

Supplements

Supplements in pregnancy are a bit like back-up singers: they're not the star of the show (you can't get everything your baby needs through them alone) but they provide valuable support. I've organized this section the way you might your medicine cabinet or your bedside table. Here are the supplements you want to have on hand during your pregnancy.

→ **A broad prenatal supplement:** This will contain many vitamins (vitamins A, B, C, D, E) and minerals (magnesium, zinc, selenium . . .). While, as mentioned, it's always best to get your vitamins and minerals from a nourishing diet, a prenatal supplement is a good insurance policy. Make sure it contains:

  → **Folate**—400mcg of folic acid (the synthetic and most widely studied form of folate used in supplements) is recommended from the moment you start trying to conceive, increasing to 600mcg during pregnancy and lowering again to 500mcg while breastfeeding. A potentially superior option to look for is methyl-folate, a form that is immediately usable by the body. It may be especially helpful for people with genetic variants that slow the conversion of folic acid, and emerging evidence suggests it could be even more effective at preventing malformations than traditional folic acid. Folate works hand in hand with choline to help neurodevelopment and cognitive outcomes in children.

→ **Vitamin D**—this nutrient supports both your immunity and your baby's growing bones. During pregnancy you need about 600IU (15mcg) per day. Oily fish like salmon (840IU per 100g serving), mackerel (400IU per 100g serving), or sardines (370IU per 100g serving) are excellent natural sources—as, of course, they are for DHA, so if you eat these fish you will get your DHA and vitamin D in one. Nevertheless, because deficiency is common worldwide, taking a supplement is a smart back-up.

→ **Iodine**—many prenatals contain around 200mcg per serving. This may not be necessary if you use iodized salt and get enough iodine from food. Think of it as an insurance policy again. It's unlikely that you will go higher than the 1,100mcg upper daily limit, but refer to the Action Plan on pages 198–200 to double-check which foods contain iodine.

→ **Choline (optional)**—if your prenatal includes choline (often as choline bitartrate), see it as a nice bonus, but food is always the better source as the absorption is superior. Aim to get your 450mg+ daily through food, and see supplements as a boost. For example, while my prenatal contained 300mg of choline bitartrate, I still aimed for 700mg of choline from food daily, and considered the supplement the top-up, not the foundation. If you don't eat any eggs, it may be helpful to add a choline supplement to make sure you get 450mg+ daily.

→ **If you don't take a broad prenatal:** make sure you have a methylated folate supplement as a minimum.

→ **Omega-3s:** As explained in Chapter 4, omega-3s, and DHA in particular, help build your baby's brain and eyes, reduce inflammation, and lower the risk of preterm birth; and 70–96 percent of moms are deficient in it. So taking a supplement is a great idea. You'll find them packaged as "omega-3 supplements," which include not only DHA but EPA as well (go to my webpage below for my recommendation). **You will want to be getting at least the recommended 300mg a day of DHA, 500mg ideally, but up to 2,000mg daily might be what you need depending on your omega-3 index level.** It's up to you and your medical team to decide how high you want to go.

→ **Iron:** Your baby draws heavily on your iron stores, especially in the third trimester. If your ferritin levels dip, your doctor will likely recommend supplementing. Of course, iron from food is still a better choice, but supplementing can be essential if levels drop too low.

→ **Protein powder:** Although not technically a "supplement," protein powder does nonetheless give you more protein than food alone. You must use one that is third-party tested for heavy metals; and ideally with no flavorings. I used unflavored whey isolate from grass-fed cows. If you are vegan, vegan protein powders exist. (See the link at the bottom of this page for my recommended protein powders.)

→ **If you breastfeed:** Take the supplements throughout.

→ **If you are on a vegan diet:** Supplements aren't optional. In order to get the building blocks necessary for your baby, you need:

- → Vitamin B12
- → Iron
- → Choline from vegan sources
- → DHA from algae
- → Vitamin D
- → Calcium
- → Zinc

To see links to my recommended supplement brands, go to glucosegoddess.com/pages/supplements-pregnancy (or scan the QR code below).

Supplement brands

For my recommended protein powders, go to glucosegoddess.com/pages/best-protein-powders (or scan the QR code below).

Protein powders

Trimester-by-trimester recap

Wow, what a journey we've been on together. I know it's a lot to take in, so in this short section I'm going to pull everything together and give you a bird's-eye view of the Action Plans. Think of it as the cheat sheet for pregnancy nutrition.

First, let's talk about calories. Over these nine months, your energy needs increase only a little: about an extra 70 calories per day in the first trimester (that's just ten almonds), an additional 260 calories in the second (an avocado), and 500 calories in the third (a small sandwich). In other words, you're not really "eating for two" . . . more like eating for one and a quarter.

What *does* rise sharply are your needs for specific nutrients. Our building blocks, and a few more. Choline. Protein. DHA. Iron. Vitamins. Minerals. These don't just creep up: they skyrocket. **Which means pregnancy isn't about piling more food on your plate—it's about putting different things on it.** The focus is not *how much* you eat, but *what* you eat.

The simplest and most powerful way to do this is to ease up on the foods that are low in nutrients and relatively high in glucose, fructose, and calories: starches such as white bread, processed flour-based products, and sugars such as breakfast cereals, fruit juice, fizzy drinks, sweets, and pastries, and to fill your plate instead with foods packed with the building blocks your baby needs: protein, choline, and iron-rich foods such as eggs, chicken, beef, beans, lentils, and dairy; DHA-rich foods like salmon, sardines, and trout; healthy fats, such as olive oil, butter, avocadoes, and nuts; and fruits and vegetables with micronutrients and vitamins like spinach, broccoli, berries, and oranges.

It's about rearranging your plate so the **building blocks are at the center.**

In case of doubt...

If you're out and about, need a quick snack, aren't sure what to order from a menu, or find yourself starving after a 4 a.m. nursing session and want to know what you should eat that will give you the most benefits—reach for some kind of animal food. Whether it's Greek yogurt, an omelet, a piece of fish, or even a hamburger (skip the side of fries), these foods always deliver protein and choline, while keeping your glucose steady.

TRIMESTER-BY-TRIMESTER RECAP

Herewith your pregnancy road map at a glance:

	Glucose	Choline	Protein	DHA
1st trimester	If you're nauseous, eat what you can stomach, even if it's just carbs. If you're *not* nauseous, keep your sugar intake minimal and use the glucose hacks to lower your spikes.	450mg/day or more (again, don't worry about achieving this if nausea makes it hard).	1.22g/kg/day ideally, but it's okay if you can't stomach any. However, note that some protein first thing in the morning can help ease nausea a little.	Supplement with omega-3s if you can: 500–1,000mg DHA daily is a good goal—but decide with your care team. Eat fish 3x a week (even one portion is good, so don't stress if this is a struggle owing to first-trimester nausea).
2nd trimester	Keep your added sugar intake as low as possible, and use the hacks to lower your spikes. You need just a little bit of extra glucose: the equivalent of a small cup of rice. Get it from starches instead of sugars.	450mg+ daily	1.52g/kg/day	Supplement with omega-3s. Eat fish 3x a week if you can.

TRIMESTER-BY-TRIMESTER RECAP

3rd trimester	Keep your added sugar intake as low as possible, and use the hacks to lower your spikes. You now need a bit more glucose: 70g/day, or 1½ cups of rice. Get your glucose from starches instead of sugars.	450mg+ daily	1.52g/kg/day	Supplement with omega-3s, and potentially stop these a little bit before your due date, depending on what your care team advises. Eat fish 3x a week if you can.
Breastfeeding	Less important, but excess sugar intake can pass into breast milk, so keep doing the hacks if you can.	550mg+ daily	1.9g/kg/day	Supplement with omega-3s. Eat fish 3x a week if you can.

And in case you find tables a little hard to use, here are the simple checklists that I used during the second and third trimesters of pregnancy and while breastfeeding to see at a glance whether I was hitting my building-block goals (during the first trimester, I was too nauseous, so I just ate what I could). You can also download an extra copy and print it out at glucosegoddess.com/ or with this QR code.

Pregnancy checklist

Pregnancy checklist

Weekly checklist
- ☐ Fish once
- ☐ Fish a second time
- ☐ Fish a third time
- ☐ Nori sheet once
- ☐ Nori sheet a second time

Daily checklist
- ☐ Savory breakfast with protein
- ☐ Did you have 4 eggs for breakfast?
- ☐ Lunch with protein
- ☐ Dinner with protein
- ☐ If you skipped eggs at breakfast, does your daily choline from your meals still add up to 450mg+?
- ☐ Avoided eating sugar on an empty stomach

Breastfeeding checklist

(This is the same checklist, but does not include "avoiding sugar on an empty stomach" as it's less important at this stage. Although of course, still good to do if you can.)

Weekly checklist
- [ ] Fish once
- [ ] Fish a second time
- [ ] Fish a third time
- [ ] Nori sheet once
- [ ] Nori sheet a second time

Daily checklist
- [ ] Savory breakfast with protein
- [ ] Did you have 4 eggs for breakfast?
- [ ] Lunch with protein
- [ ] Dinner with protein
- [ ] If you skipped eggs at breakfast, does your daily choline from your meals still add up to 450mg+?

Sample meal plans

And finally, to help you turn the checklists into real meals, here's a glimpse of a typical day on my plate. Eggs were my daily staple—nature's richest source of choline and an easy way to meet my needs. But in case eggs aren't your thing, I've also created an alternative menu, free of both eggs and meat, to show how you can still cover your protein and choline requirements with fewer animal foods. You can find the recipes I used here in the recipe section at the end of the book.

Example meal plan: with eggs

Breakfast: 4 Parmesan Fried Eggs (page 288)
- ✓ 46g protein (out of my personal 106g daily goal in the second and third trimesters)
- ✓ 565mg choline (daily goal achieved)
- ✓ 120mg DHA (from the eggs)

Lunch: 4 Salmon and Feta Fishcakes (page 296), side of rice, five squares of dark chocolate as dessert
- ✓ 41g protein
- ✓ 185mg choline
- ✓ 1,960mg DHA
- ✓ One out of three portions of weekly fish
- ✓ Sugar after a meal, not on an empty stomach

Afternoon snack: Yogurt bowl with protein powder, nut butter, and fruit ("My Absolute Favorite Snack," page 304)
- ✓ 58g protein
- ✓ 115mg choline

Dinner: Store-bought tomato soup with a nori sheet broken into it and half a shredded chicken breast, side of pasta, and some Chocolate Bark with nuts and seeds (page 322)
- ✓ 18g protein
- ✓ 58mg choline
- ✓ One of two weekly nori sheets
- ✓ Sugar after a meal, not on an empty stomach

Total for the day:
- ✓ 163g protein (higher than my 106g daily goal in the second and third trimesters)
- ✓ 923mg choline (beyond the 450mg+ goal)
- ✓ One of three weekly portions of oily fish
- ✓ One of two weekly nori sheets
- ✓ Sugar as dessert, not on an empty stomach

Example meal plan: without eggs (and without meat)

Breakfast: Yogurt bowl with protein powder, nut butter, and fruit ("My Absolute Favorite Snack", page 304)
- ✓ 58g protein
- ✓ 115mg choline

Lunch: 4 Salmon and Feta Fishcakes (page 296), side of rice, five squares of dark chocolate as dessert
- ✓ 41g protein
- ✓ 185mg choline
- ✓ 1,960mg DHA
- ✓ One of three portions of weekly fish
- ✓ Sugar after a meal, not on an empty stomach

Afternoon snack: Crispy Chickpeas (page 308)
- ✓ 7g protein
- ✓ 15mg choline

Dinner: Store-bought tomato soup with a nori sheet broken into it, 200g of baked tempeh, zucchini salad with 60g crumbled feta, some Chocolate Bark with nuts and seeds (page 322):
- ✓ 54g protein
- ✓ 100mg choline
- ✓ One of two weekly nori sheets
- ✓ Sugar after a meal, not on an empty stomach

Total for the day:
- ✓ 160g protein (higher than my 106g daily goal in the second and third trimesters)
- ✓ 415mg choline (just under the 450mg+ goal; adding a choline supplement will get you higher)
- ✓ One of three portions of weekly fish
- ✓ One of two weekly nori sheets
- ✓ Sugar as dessert, not on an empty stomach

All the best

When I was pregnant, I carried wishes for my son like small prayers. I thought: I hope he gets his dad's strong muscles, but not his midnight love affair with Haribo sweets. I hope he doesn't edge toward prediabetes like I did in my twenties, or wrestle with the shadows of mental health that I've known. I hope he's sharp as a tack, quick to laugh, and I really, *really* hope he escapes the cancers that have devastated a branch of our family.

If I hadn't come across the science that I have shared in this book, I would have thought that all I could do was that: Hope. Wish. Cross my fingers. But now I know better. A child's health outcomes are not just a case of: "It runs in the family." By changing what I ate during these nine months, I had an opportunity to shift the odds. And you can too.

As you've learned throughout these pages, a pregnancy diet isn't just calories in and kilograms on. It's the soil from which your baby grows. It shapes the scaffolding of his brain, the strength of his organs, the set point of his hormones, and the blueprint of his metabolism. It even epigenetically programs his DNA toward or away from disease.

With how you eat, you have the chance to reduce his risk of prematurity, to lower his risk of diabetes, asthma, and sugar addiction, to boost his cognitive development, and more. In the span of a lifetime, these nine months may feel short (though at the time, they may not!), but they are profoundly powerful. They are your opportunity to give your baby the four building blocks of pregnancy nutrition—steady glucose, and enough choline, protein, DHA—as well as iron, vitamins, and minerals. Not only to grow day by day, but to carry a foundation of health for life.

You don't need perfection. But every egg you eat for choline, every salmon fillet for DHA, every extra 30g of protein at breakfast, every time you save sweet foods for after a meal instead of before—these are not small acts. They're instructions to your baby's DNA, postcards to the womb, shaping how durable his organs will be, how his metabolism will respond to sugar, how well his neurons will connect . . . quite simply, how he will meet the world.

The science is clear: pregnancy nutrition can help explain why two children can share the same classroom, yet one soaks up knowledge while the other struggles. Why two people can eat the same diet, but one develops diabetes and the other doesn't. Why two can train the same way in the gym, yet only one builds muscle. Why two can face the same challenges, but have different mental health outcomes.

I thought about this the night my son was born. I didn't sleep at all; I just stared at him, wondering what his life would be like. I can't know, nor can I control, how it will unfold—what he'll face, where he'll go, who he'll love, and how happy he will be. I can only hope. Wish. Cross my fingers.

But there is one thing I do know: by putting this research into practice, I've given him a gift. A foundation for health that may help him thrive a little more easily, weather hardship with greater strength, and step into the world with a bit more resilience.

To carry a baby for these nine months is, indeed, a responsibility. And I don't know about you, but instead of this science making me feel pressured, it helped me navigate that responsibility with more confidence.

My boy was never just a bun in the oven. He was a little tree—rooted in my best effort at providing a great soil—now off to grow taller and stronger than me.

I hope what you've learned in these pages gives you power, agency, and a clear plan forward. Wishing you and your baby all the very best.

With love,
Jessie

Thank you

Thank you to the scientists and researchers whose work fills these pages. I hope I've done your discoveries justice.

Elissa, thank you for your generosity toward me in this life, which I don't quite know how I've deserved, and for your exceptional scientific review. Aurea, I am endlessly grateful for your commitment to my books—there is truly no one I'd rather spend a month unraveling and rebuilding the structure of the protein chapter with. Susanna, thank you for the diving board you built for me, from which I've been able to leap again and again. Emily, thank you for bringing your sharp pen and hawk eye to these pages. Faustine, Justine, Annie, Emma, Alex, and Judy, thank you for your precious contributions.

To my dearest husband: you are my everything. Thank you for being as gifted at supporting me through my work and existential breakdowns as you are at feeding me the most delicious food every day.

And finally to my incredible sunshine of a son, thank you for choosing me to be your mom. I carried you with all my heart; and I promise, I ate a shit ton of eggs.

Scientific references

If you'd like to dive deeper into the science behind this book, you can. To save paper, to reduce the weight of this book for shipping, and to make sure you always have the most up-to-date links, I've gathered the 600 scientific references I used to write this book in one place.

You can find them at glucosegoddess.com/pages/science-pregnancy, or simply scan the QR code below.

Index

active phase of labor, 233
acute inflammation, 69
adenosine, 216
adenosine triphosphate (ATP), 32
ADHD in children
    correlation with gestational diabetes, 67, 68
    correlation with low choline levels, 109, 110
    correlation with type 1 diabetes, 68
    and preterm birth, 183
ALA, 203–4
alcohol, 212–14
algae-based omega-3 supplements, 198
allergies, 189–90, 247
American Academy of Pediatrics (AAP), 103
American College of Obstetricians and Gynecologists, 217
Amino Acid Response (AAR) pathway, 145
amino acids, 126, 127, 169–71

animal-based proteins, 160
anthocyanins, 218
antibodies, 126
Anti-Spike Formula, 87
arginine, 169
asthma, 189, 190
attention, 97
autism, 67–68

baby formula
    choline in, 117, 123–24, 248
    choosing, 248
    DHA in, 187, 200
    ingredients in, 248
    protein in, 133
Barker, David J., 134–37, 151
baseline glucose levels
    high levels, 36
    ideal levels, 36
    in low birth weight babies, 136
    shifts during pregnancy, 37–40
    tests and results, 90
BDNF (brain-derived-neurotrophic factor), 175, 207–9

INDEX

behavioral difficulties. *See also* ADHD
  correlation with gestational diabetes, 67
  correlation with low DHA levels, 179
birth comb, 244
birth plan, 227
birth stories, 231, 240–43
birth weight
  low, and caffeine, 216
  low, genetic causes of, 148
  low, health consequences, 134–40, 149
  normal, weight range for, 49
bloodstream, 26–28
blood sugar crashes, 24
blood tests and results, 90–93
BMI (Body Mass Index), 157
body weight, studies on, 49–50
brain development
  BDNF for, 207–9
  in breastfed babies, 246, 247
  choline for, 97–98
  DHA for, 176, 178–80
  impact of alcohol on, 212–14
  impact of glucose on, 65–70
  impact of inflammation on, 65–70
  and maternal exercise, 207–11
  neuron growth during, 174
  protein for, 139
  in third trimester, 64
breakfast, skipping, 81
breakfasts, savory, 76–81
breast cancer, 136

breastfeeding
  and alcohol, 214
  and caffeine, 217
  checklist, 258
  choline needs, 104, 117, 118
  DHA needs, 187–88, 195–96, 200, 202
  effect on baby's DNA, 57–58
  iodine needs, 202
  muscle loss during, 143
  nutrition road map, 256
  protein needs, 132, 157, 163–64, 165
  sample protein meals, 163–64
  studies on, 247
  vitamin B12 needs, 154
breast milk
  adaptability of, 246–47
  alcohol in, 214
  caffeine in, 217
  choline in, 117
  DHA in, 187
  effect on baby's DNA, 47–58
  health benefits for baby, 246–48
  proteins in, 143
  RNAs in, 57, 246
  sugars in, 64
  vitamin B12 in, 154
broccoli, 218

caffeine, 215–17
calories, 247–48, 253
cancer, 136

INDEX

carbohydrates (carbs). *See also* starches; sugar
  broken down into glucose, 33
  reducing nausea with, 24
carotenoids, 218
Centers for Disease Control (CDC), 214
cervix, 182, 233–34
childbirth, 225–45
  author's birth story, 240–43
  best positions, 235–36
  continuous support during, 225–27
  first stage, 233–36
  medical interventions, 239
  pain management and labor kit, 244–45
  reducing fear of, 230–32
  second and third stages, 237–38
  speeding up labor, 228–29
  top tips, 235
chlorophylls, 218
cholesterol, 116–17, 120–21
choline, 96–124
  action plan, 113–17
  adding to diet, 116–17
  animal studies on, 102–3
  in baby formula, 117, 123–24, 248
  biological role, 97–98
  for brain development, 97–98
  for breastfeeding, 104, 117, 118
  in breast milk, 117
  in eggs, 106–7, 116–17
  food sources, 114–15
  frequently asked questions, 120–24
  impact on epigenetic programming, 98
  impact on memory, 97, 100, 101, 109
  in liver, 105
  low, impact on mother, 101
  measuring, 113–16
  in protein-rich foods, 152–53
  for quick snacks, 254
  recap, for pregnancy and breastfeeding, 118
  recommended intake, 104
  statistics on, 104–5, 111–12
  studies on, 100–101, 108–11
  supplements, 111, 117, 122, 123, 250–51
  top tips, 119
  upper limits, 108, 124
  in vegan diet, 122
choline bitartrate, 250
chronic inflammation, 35, 69
cigarettes, 106
coffee and tea, 215–17
cognition, 109, 178–79, 183
collagen, 126, 155, 220
concentration, 101
continuous glucose monitor (CGM), 34, 88
contractions, 182, 234–35, 237
C-reactive protein (CRP), 67, 69, 91
C-reactive protein (CRP) test, 65, 185
C-sections, 225–26, 239

INDEX

dairy, 80, 191–92, 199
dates, 89, 228–29
Da Vinci, Leonardo, 26
depression, 210
developmental delays, 247
DHA
  action plan, 193–98
  in baby formula, 248
  biological function, 175–76
  deficiency, consequences of, 178–80
  deficiency, prevalence of, 184
  food sources, 175, 194–96
  frequently asked questions, 203–5
  in omega-3 supplements, 186–88, 189–90, 196–98, 251
  recap, for pregnancy and breastfeeding, 202
  recommendations on, 176–77, 184
  reducing allergy risk with, 189–90
  safe upper limits, 188
  target daily goal, 193
  target weekly goal, 194
  top tips, 202–3
  transferred to baby, 182–83
  vegan options, 203–4
diabetes. *See also* gestational diabetes; type 2 diabetes
  correlation with psychiatric disorders, 66–70
  IGF2 gene linked to, 145
  minimizing risk, with breastfeeding, 247
  type 1, 68

dilation, 233–34
DNA
  contained in sperm, 18
  epigenetic programming, 55–59, 63, 98, 145, 246
dopamine, 60, 61–62, 63–64
doulas, 225–26
Dutch famine, 135–36, 144, 145
dyslexia, 109

eczema, 189, 221
effacement, 233–34
eggs (dietary)
  adding to diet, 120
  and cholesterol, 120–21
  choline in, 106–7, 116–17
  DHA in, 195
  undercooked, 121–22
eggs (in uterus), 18
elastin, 127, 155
embryo, 19, 20
endorphins, 244
EPA, 188, 251
epigenetic programming
  choline required for, 98
  in Dutch famine babies, 145
  of fat-storage and fat-burning genes, 56–57
  of genes linked to diabetes, 55
  influencing, 58–59
  of leptin gene, 55, 57–58
  for sugar cravings, 63
  through breast milk, 57–58, 246

INDEX

European Food Safety Authority, 217
exercise, 207–11

fasting glucose levels, 36, 90. *See also* baseline glucose level
fat-burning genes, 56–57
fat cells, 35, 48
fat mass, 35, 48, 148
fats, dietary, 75, 77
fat-storage genes, 56–57, 139
fermented foods, 221–22
ferritin, 153–54, 251
Fetal Alcohol Syndrome (FAS), 213
fetal growth restriction (FGR), 149–50
fetal programming, 58, 135
fetus
    cell division, 96–97
    glucose requirements, 42
    impact of glucose on, 48
    ribosome activity, 128–29
    signs of growth restriction, 150
fiber
    food sources of, 75
    in fresh whole fruit, 71
    impact on glucose absorption, 36
    impact on microbiome, 219
first trimester
    caffeine during, 215
    caloric needs, 253
    choline needs, 118
    DHA and iodine needs, 202
    minimizing sugar intake, 86
    nutritional needs, 20–25
    nutrition road map, 255
    protein needs, 130–31, 157, 165
fish, 194–95, 199
folate, 99, 249–50
folic acid, 249
folic-acid deficiency, 100
food allergies, 189–90, 247
food preferences, in babies, 220
fructose, 36, 42, 63
fruits
    fiber in, 36, 71
    nutritional benefits, 218–19
    reducing sugar cravings with, 76

GDF15 hormone, 23
gestational diabetes
    addressing, with exercise, 210
    addressing, with omega-3 supplements, 187
    causes of, 45
    description of, 43
    impact on mother's muscles, 142
    from low choline, 101
    statistics on, 148
    studies on, 45
    test for, 44–47, 91–93
gestational diabetes (impact on babies)
    increased risk of autism, 67
    increased risk of diabetes, 48–50, 56
    increased risk of low birth weight, 134, 136, 139
    increased risk of psychiatric disorders, 66–70

INDEX

ginger nausea gummies, 23
glucose, 33–93. *See also* glucose spikes
  biological function, 33
  effect on baby's DNA, 63
  excess, effect on metabolism, 147
  excess, stored in body, 35, 48
  food chart, 75
  frequently asked questions, 80–81, 87–89
  low, triggering nausea, 24
  needed by the placenta, 41
  recap, for pregnancy and breastfeeding, 86
  from starches and sugars, 33
  testing for gestational diabetes, 44–47, 91–93
  top tips for, 87
  transferred to fetus, 41
Glucose Challenge Test (GCT), 92
glucose levels, baseline (fasting)
  blood tests and results, 36, 90
  in low birth weight babies, 136
  shifts during pregnancy, 37–40
Glucose Revolution (Inchauspé), 33
glucose spikes
  consequences of, 35–36
  defined, 34
  from eating dates, 228–29
  impact on inflammation, 66
  minimizing, tips for, 81–85
  during pregnancy, 38–40
Greek yogurt, 24–25
gummies, nausea, 23

hCG hormone, 21–23
heart disease, 134, 136
heart rate, 209
hemoglobin, 126
high blood pressure, 139
hip muscle strength, 141
HOMA-IR ratio, 90–91
hunger signals, 139
hyperemesis gravidarum, 23

IGF2 gene, 145
immune system, strengthening
  with breast milk, 246
  with DHA, 189–90
  with probiotics, 221
Indicator Amino Acid Oxidation Method (IAAO), 130–33
inflammation
  acute, 69
  chronic, 69
  from glucose spikes, 35
  impact on brain development, 65–70
  link to immune responses, 189–90
  measuring, 185
  from omega-6s, 181–83
  reducing, with omega-3s, 181
  sugar-induced, 190
insulin, 35, 126
insulin resistance
  measuring, 90–91
  in newborns, 48
  throughout pregnancy, 38–40

INDEX

intrauterine growth restriction (IUGR), 149–50
iodine
  daily goal, 198–200
  food sources, 199
  recap, for pregnancy and breastfeeding, 202
  safe upper limit, 192, 200
  supplements, 250
  for thyroid hormones, 191
iodized salt, 192, 199
IQ
  and DHA levels, 178, 179
  and high choline levels, 109
  and iodine levels, 191
  and preterm births, 183
iron, 153–54, 251

kefir, 222
kimchi, 222

labor, 225–45
  active phase, 233
  author's birth story, 240–43
  best positions, 235–36
  continuous support during, 225–27
  first stages of, 233–36
  labor kit, 245
  latent phase, 233
  medical interventions, 239
  pain management, 244–45
  reducing fear of, 230–32
  second and third stages, 237–38
  speeding up, 228–29
  top tips, 235
latent phase of labor, 233
learning, and choline, 97
LEP gene, 55
leptin hormone, 55, 57–58
liver, 101, 105
low birth weight
  and caffeine, 216
  genetic causes of, 148
  health consequences, 134–40, 149
lung development, 190

meal plans, sample, 259–61
memory, and choline, 97, 100, 101, 109
mental health, 106
mercury, in fish, 195
metabolism, 139, 147
methyl-folate, 249
methyl groups, 98
microalgae, 175
microbiome
  effect on immune system, 221–22
  effect on inflammation, 219–20
  seeding, with breast milk, 246
  seeding, with skin-to-skin contact, 237–38
  seeding, with vaginal fluids, 239
microglia, 65–66
micronutrients, 218–19
microplastics, 223–24
midwives, 225–26
milk, dairy, 80

minerals, 218–19
miscarriages, 11–13, 215
mitochondria, 32
morning sickness, 79–80
muscles
   protein breakdown in, 141–45
   weakened, from low choline levels, 101
   weakened by breastfeeding, 143

natto, 222
nausea
   causes of, 21–23
   morning sickness, 79–80
   tips for, 23–25
neural tube, 97
neural tube defects, 100
neurodevelopmental impairments, 68, 183
neurons, 97
neurotransmitters, 97
Nitrogen Balance Technique, 130
nori sheets, 192
nucleus accumbens, 61

obesity
   correlation with low birth weight, 136
   correlation with maternal glucose levels, 52
   and Dutch famine babies, 49–50
   IGF2 gene linked to, 145
   impact of breastfeeding on, 58, 247
ocular development, 178

oily fish, 194–95
omega-3 index, 185–86
omega-3s. *See also* DHA
   effect on preterm births, 183–84
   foods rich in, 182
   reducing inflammation with, 181
   supplements, 186–88, 189–90, 196–98, 251
   testing for, 185–86
omega-6s, 181–83, 200–201
Oral Glucose Tolerance Test (OGTT), 44, 92
organ meats, 105
overnight fasting, 24
oxygen, 32, 210–11
oxytocin
   inhibited by stress hormones, 230
   released in skin-to-skin contact, 238
   role in labor and childbirth, 226
   for uterine contractions, 233

pain management, 235, 244–45
pasteurized eggs, 122
phytonutrients, 218–19
pitocin, 227
placenta
   after childbirth, 238
   biological role, 26–28, 128
   glucose requirements, 41
   protein-restricted, 140
   underperforming, 144
plant-based proteins, 160
plastics, 223–24

INDEX

postpartum, 142
prediabetes, 36, 47, 49–50
preeclampsia, 101
pregnancy. *See also* first trimester;
    second trimester; third trimester
  checklist, 257
  choline-rich liver for, 105
  first week of, 19
  muscle loss in, 141–45
  road map, 255–56
pregnancy loss, 11–15
prenatal supplements
  with choline, 123, 250–51
  with folate, 249–50
  with iodine, 250
  lack of omega-3s in, 196
  micronutrients in, 219
  with vitamin B12, 154
  with vitamin D, 250
prenatal vitamins, 117
preterm birth, 182–84
probiotics, 221–22
prostaglandins, 182, 239
protein, 126–71
  action plan, 156–64
  adding to diet, 129, 161–64
  biological function, 126–27
  at breakfast, 77
  in breast milk, 143
  calculating, table for, 157–59
  calculating need for, 156–57
  complete, 160, 170–71
  food sources of, 75, 127, 158–59
  formed during pregnancy, 128
  frequently asked questions, 167–68
  health benefits of, 152–55
  incomplete, 160
  in muscles, 141–42
  plant sources of, 170–71
  for quick snacks, 254
  recap, for pregnancy and
    breastfeeding, 165
  reducing nausea with, 23
  required for pregnancy, 130–33
  restricted, health consequences,
    146–50
  restricted, statistics on, 132–33
  top tips for, 165–66
  upper safe limits, 167
protein leverage hypothesis, 152
protein powder, 162, 167, 170,
  251–52
psychiatric disorders, 66–70

resistance training, 210
retinas, 178
ribosomes, 127
RNAs, in breast milk, 57, 246

salmonella, 121
salt, 192, 199
sauerkraut, 222
schizophrenia, 66, 110, 136
seafood, 175–76. *See also* fish
seaweed, 191
second trimester
  caloric needs, 253
  choline needs, 118

275

INDEX

second trimester (*cont.*)
   DHA and iodine needs, 202
   glucose needs, 86
   nutrition road map, 255
   protein needs, 130–31, 157, 165
   what happens during, 26–29
"sick quitter effect," 212
"silent" miscarriages, 11–13
skin-to-skin contact, 237–38
snacks, 24
sperm, 18
starches
   choosing, over sugar, 74
   containing glucose, 75
   molecules in, 36
   reducing nausea with, 25
   in third trimester, 42
stress hormones, 230
stretch marks, 220
sugar. *See also* glucose
   action plan, 71–85
   and asthma, 190
   containing glucose and fructose, 75
   cravings for, 60–64
   and food allergies, 190
   foods containing, 71–72, 75
   foods with 25g of, 74
   impact on baby's DNA, 56–59
   minimizing glucose spikes from, 81–85
   molecules in, 36
   UK rationing studies, 51–53
   WHO recommendation on, 53, 73

supplements. *See also* prenatal supplements
   choline, 111, 117, 122, 123, 250–51
   iron, 251
   omega-3s, 186–88, 189–90, 196–98, 251
   recommended brands, 252
   for vegans, 252
sweeteners, 80

tea and coffee, 215–17
teenagers, 49
teratogen, 213
third trimester
   brain development, 64
   caffeine and, 215
   caloric needs, 253
   choline needs, 118
   decline in physical function, 210
   DHA and iodine needs, 202
   glucose needs, 42
   minimizing sugar intake, 86
   nutrition roadmap, 256
   protein needs, 130–31, 157, 165
   what happens during, 26–29
thrifty phenotype hypothesis, 137
thyroid hormones, 191, 192
triplets, 133
twins, 133
type 1 diabetes, 68
type 2 diabetes
   correlation with maternal glucose, 51–52

glucose test numbers, 36
link with low birth weight, 134, 136
studies on, 49–50

ultra-processed foods, 200
ultrasounds, 150
US Institute of Medicine, 104
uterine milk, 20
uterine secretions, 98

vaginal seeding, 239
vegan diet
  algae-based omega-3 supplements for, 198
  amino acid refresher for, 169–71
  choline supplements for, 122
  conversion of ALA to DHA, 203–4
  plant-based proteins for, 168, 169–71
  required vitamins and minerals, 252
  vitamin B12 for, 154–55
vegetables, 77, 218–20
vegetarian diet, 149, 154, 167
vinegar, 87
vitamin A, 105
vitamin B12, 154–55
vitamin C, 99, 220
vitamin D, 250
vitamins
  prenatal, 117
  in vegetables and fruits, 218–19
VTA (ventral tegmental area), 60–61

World Health Organization (WHO)
  recommendation on alcohol, 214
  recommendation on exercise, 211
  recommendation on sugar, 53, 73

yogurt, 24–25, 222
yolk sac, 20

About the author

Jessie Inchauspé is a French biochemist, founder, and internationally bestselling author. She has devoted her career to translating cutting-edge science into easy tips to help people improve their physical and mental health. Through her books *Glucose Revolution* and *The Glucose Goddess Method*, which have sold more than 3 million copies in 43 languages, she has reshaped the global conversation around blood sugar. Jessie is the founder of the wildly popular social community @GlucoseGoddess, where she reaches more than seven million people across platforms. She holds a BSc in mathematics from King's College, London, and an MSc in biochemistry from Georgetown University.

RECIPES

Ready to put this science into practice? Over the following pages, you'll find a collection of my go-to pregnancy recipes. They're designed to be as easy to make as they are nourishing. Each one is developed around the building blocks in this book, with several purposes in one: steadying your glucose, covering key nutrients like choline and DHA, allowing you to hit your protein target, and making consistency effortless.

First, **savory breakfasts**. Starting the day with a savory meal has multiple benefits: it steadies your glucose, jump-starts your protein intake, and offers the perfect opportunity to get a good dose of choline. Eggs make this especially easy—but if you don't eat eggs, I've included options without them that still deliver both protein and choline. And, of course, if your mornings are rushed and you prefer a no-cook start, my own go-to was My Absolute Favorite Snack on page 304.

Next come five **main dishes for lunch or dinner**. Each of these gives you at least 30g of protein, and the salmon recipes in particular will help you stay on track with DHA. You may notice that darker-colored vegetables also feature prominently. These are the ones that tend to contain more nutrients—especially antioxidants, vitamins, and minerals—so don't skimp on these. Indeed, feel free to add more of them wherever you can.

For when you're feeling hungry between meals, you'll find five **high-protein snacks**—especially helpful in the third trimester when your hunger intensifies, but your stomach reduces in size. Each one will keep your glucose steady and will keep you feeling full. I have also included a recipe with nori sheets to boost iodine.

For when you're craving **sweet things**, I've made five fruit-based or lower-sugar desserts designed to minimize your glucose spikes. They follow the "clothes on carbs" principle: sugar always paired with protein, fat, or fiber to soften the impact on your glucose levels while still giving you the dopamine hit you're after. (And if sometimes you just want a proper cookie, of course, that's fine too.)

Pick from these recipes and you'll be well on your way to creating a great soil for your baby to thrive in.

SAVORY BREAKFASTS

Mackerel Mash of Goodness

When it comes to bread during pregnancy, the winner is sourdough. The fermentation process changes the starch chains so that they create a smaller glucose spike. For a protein and omega-3 boost, I love using smoked mackerel, but you can easily swap in good-quality tinned sardines in olive oil, or even salmon, if you prefer. You can also skip the nuts and even the avocado. Think of this as a flexible template to adapt to your taste.

SERVES: 1

1 egg
1 ripe avocado
4½ oz (125g) smoked mackerel or sardine fillets
3 tbsps pasteurized cottage cheese
2 small slices of sourdough toast
¼ cup (25g) walnuts, pecans, or mixed seeds, toasted
a spoonful of pasteurized sauerkraut (optional), to serve
lemon wedges (optional), to serve
salt and freshly ground black pepper

PER PORTION (THE WHOLE RECIPE): ✓ 49g protein ✓ 270mg choline ✓ 1,090mg DHA (1,120mg if you use a free-range pasture-raised egg)

- Boil the **egg** for 10 minutes, until just hard-boiled, then drain and plunge the egg into ice water to stop the cooking.

- Cut the **avocado** flesh into rough chunks, tip them into a medium bowl, and lightly mash them with a fork.

- Skin the **mackerel or sardine fillets** and flake the flesh into the bowl. Add the **cottage cheese**, season with **salt** and **pepper**, and mix to combine.

- Pile the avocado smash onto the toasted sourdough and scatter the toasted **nuts or seeds**. Serve with a spoonful of **sauerkraut**, if you like, and wedges of **lemon** on the side.

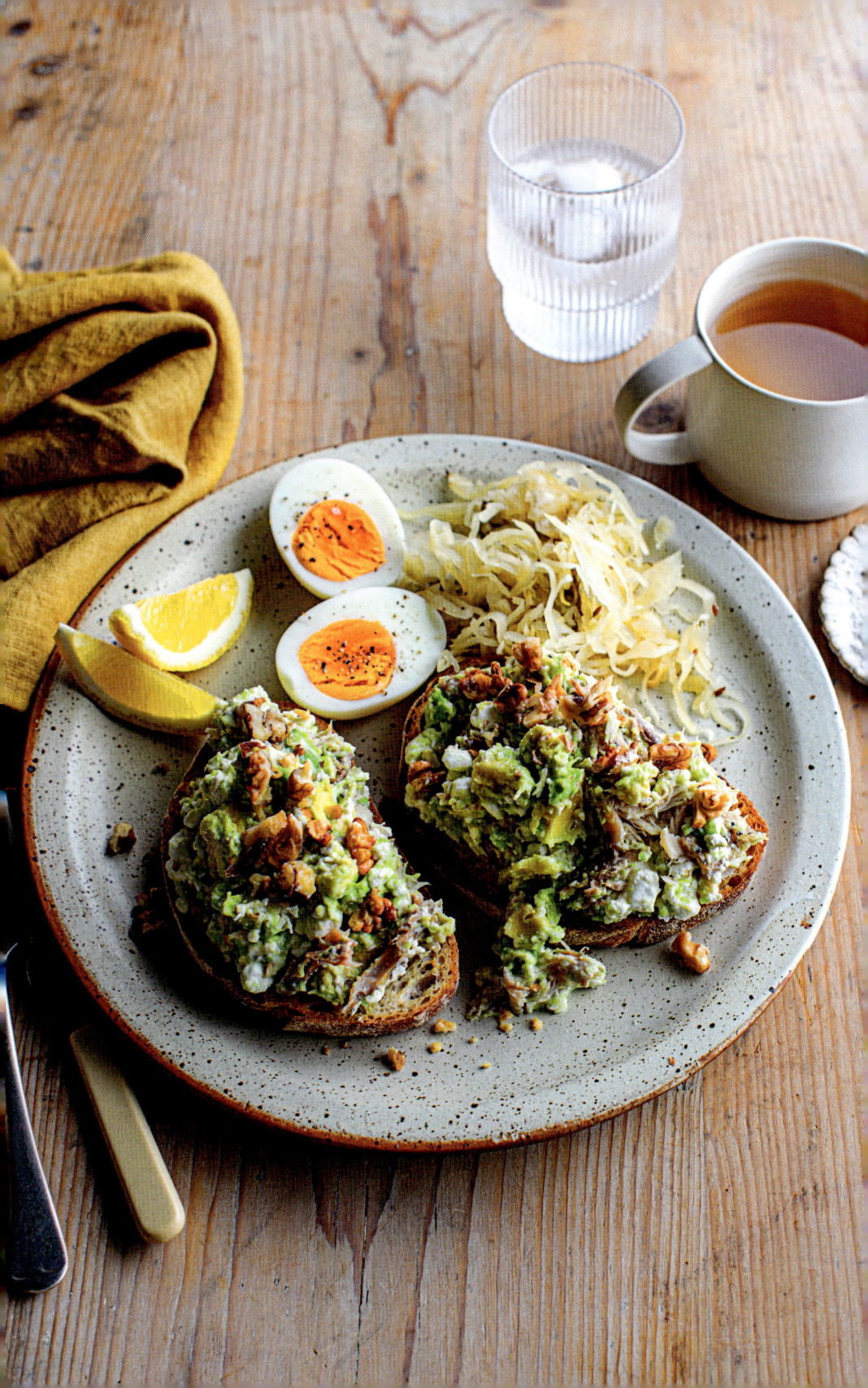

Building Blocks Frittata

This recipe is loaded with building blocks. And the best part? It makes two portions. Once it's cooked, just slice it in half—you've got breakfast for today and another serving to stash in the fridge for a few days later.

SERVES: 2

juice of ½ lemon
7 oz (200g) salmon or trout fillet
2 small zucchini
2 tbsps olive oil
8 large eggs

Scant ½ cup (100g) cottage cheese or cream cheese
½ cup (75g) frozen peas, defrosted
1 tbsp chopped dill or snipped chives
salt and freshly ground black pepper

PER PORTION (HALF THE RECIPE): ✓ 60g protein ✓ 635mg choline
✓ 1,460mg DHA (1,580mg if you use free-range pasture-raised eggs)

• Fill a small pan with water, add the **lemon juice** and a pinch of salt, and bring the water to a simmer. Place the **salmon or trout fillet** in the liquid, cover with a lid, and poach for 5–7 minutes, then remove the cooked fillet and put it aside.

• Cut the **zucchini** into slices just under ¼ inch (5mm) thick, tip the slices into a large frying pan, and add the **olive oil**. Cook the zucchini over medium heat, stirring often, for 3–4 minutes, until starting to soften.

• Meanwhile, in a medium bowl, whisk the **eggs** with the **cottage cheese** until thoroughly combined. Add the **peas** and **dill or chives** and season well with **salt** and **pepper**.

• Heat the broiler to high.

• Pour the egg mixture into the pan, around and over the vegetables. Flake the cooked fish into chunks and scatter the chunks evenly over the eggs.

• Cook the frittata on the stovetop over medium-low heat, without stirring, for about 4 minutes, until the egg has set around the edges and the middle is still liquid. Slide the pan under the hot broiler and cook for about 4 minutes more, until the egg is golden and bubbly and has completely set.

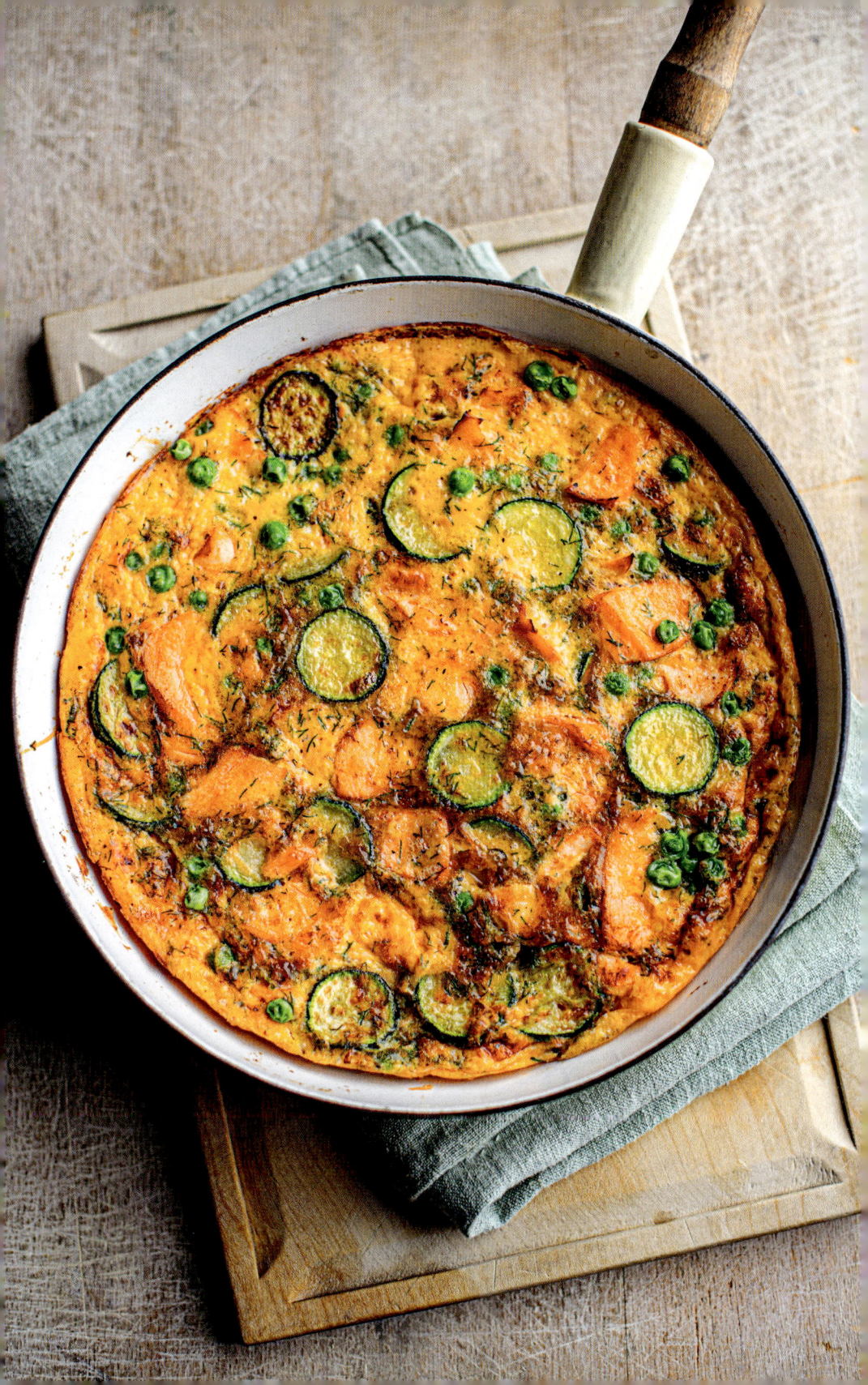

Cheesy Corn Pancakes

Okay, confession: this isn't the breakfast with the most building blocks. But some mornings just call for pancakes. Just catch up later in the day with some high-protein and choline-rich foods to hit your goals.

MAKES: 12 PANCAKES/3 PORTIONS

4 oz (100g) Brussels sprouts or collard greens, trimmed
1 cup (165g) corn kernels (either frozen and defrosted, drained from a can, or from 1½ cobs of fresh corn)
2¼ oz (65g) Gruyère cheese, grated (about ⅔ cup)

⅔ cup (75g) all-purpose flour
1 tsp baking powder
⅔ cup (160ml) whole milk
1 large egg, plus 1 large yolk
¼ cup (35g) hemp seeds
olive oil
salt and freshly ground black pepper

PER PORTION (WITHOUT OPTIONAL EXTRAS): ✓ 18g protein ✓ 115mg choline ✓ 20mg DHA (if you use free-range pasture-raised eggs)

- Slice the **Brussels sprouts or collard greens** into fine shreds, tip them into a large bowl, add the **corn kernels** and **Gruyère cheese,** and mix to combine.

- In another bowl, combine the **flour, baking powder, milk,** and whole **egg** and **yolk.** Sprinkle with **salt** and **pepper** and whisk until smooth. Add the **hemp seeds** and whisk again to incorporate them evenly into the batter. Pour the batter into the veggies and mix to thoroughly combine.

- Heat a little **olive oil** in a large frying pan over medium heat. Spoon 4 mounds of the pancake mixture into the pan—allowing a rounded large spoonful of the mixture per pancake. Cook for about 1 minute, until the batter has set around the edges, the underside is golden, and the batter on the top is starting to dry. Using a spatula, carefully flip the pancakes over and cook the other side for another 1 minute or until golden brown.

- Remove the pancakes from the pan and keep them warm on a covered serving dish while you cook the remaining mixture, adding a little more olive oil to the frying pan as needed.

- To serve, you can keep it simple with a spoonful of yogurt or sour cream, maybe a drizzle of chile oil. Or go big: blistered cherry tomatoes, sliced avocado, crispy bacon. If you're only eating one portion, keep the extras in the fridge and you'll have a couple of grab-and-go breakfasts for the week.

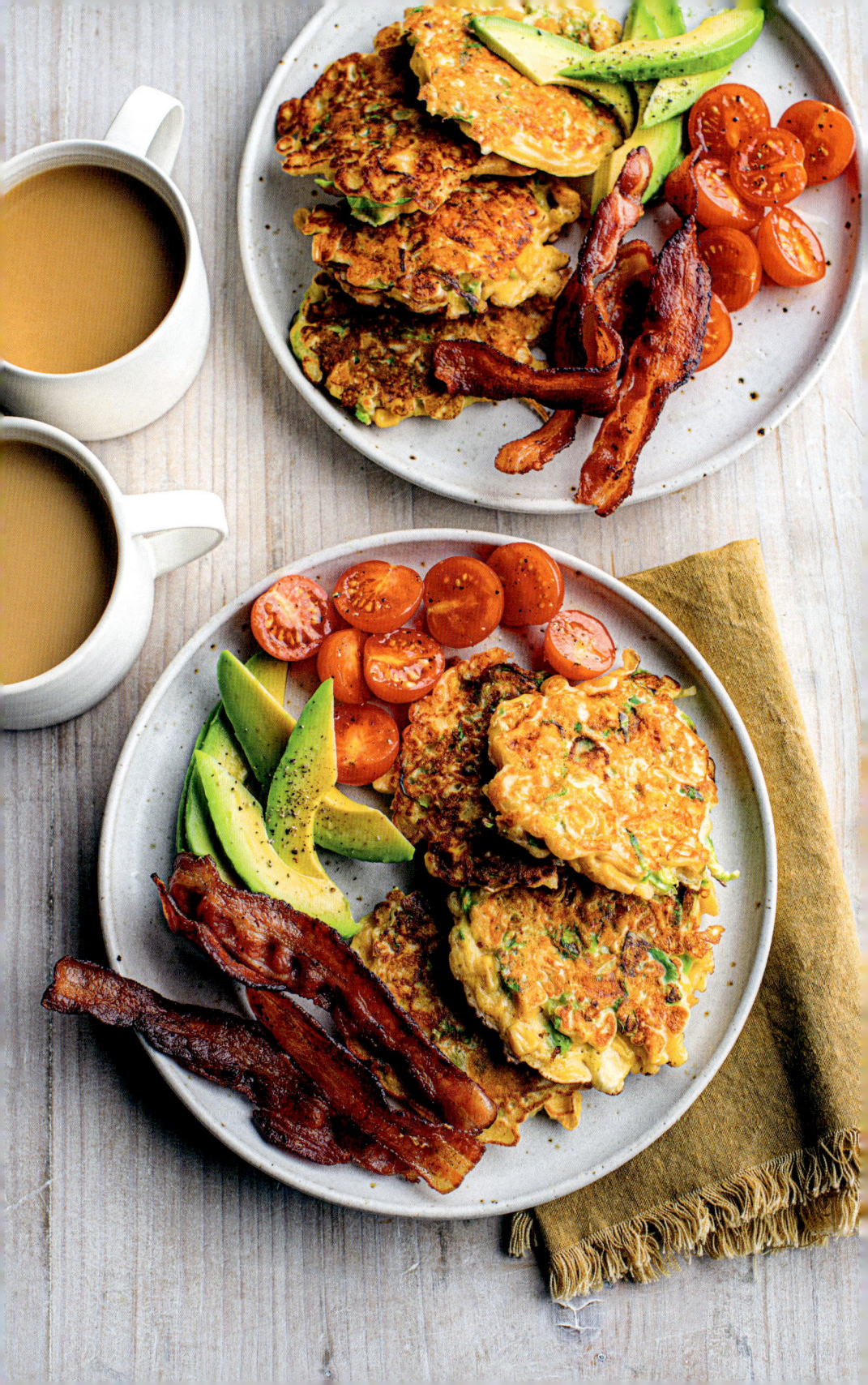

Parmesan Fried Eggs

If you've read my other books, you already know about my parmesan obsession. So, you can imagine my relief when I found out it's totally fine to eat during pregnancy. And it's also packed with protein. Yay indeed. So . . . please welcome my latest creation: parmesan fried eggs!

SERVES: 1

4 oz (120g) broccoli
½ fresh green chile
juice of ½ lime
salt and freshly ground black pepper
4 large eggs
4 rounded tbsps (75g) freshly grated parmesan
2 tsps olive oil
½ tsp za'atar, to serve (optional)

PER PORTION (THE WHOLE RECIPE): ✓ 46g protein ✓ 565mg choline ✓ 120mg DHA (if you use free-range pasture-raised eggs)

- Cut the **broccoli** into slivers and tip it into a bowl. Finely chop the **chile** and add it to the bowl with the broccoli. Squeeze in the **lime juice** and season well with **salt** and **pepper**. Mix to combine, then set aside for 10 minutes for the flavors to mingle.

- Crack each **egg** separately into its own small bowl or ramekin.

- Spoon the **parmesan** into 4 mounds in a large nonstick frying pan, then spread each mound into a 4-inch (10cm) circle. Set the pan over medium heat for 20 seconds, until the cheese just starts to melt.

- Carefully tip one **egg** on top of each mound of cheese in the pan, season with **pepper**, and cook for 30 seconds, until the edges start to set.

- Drizzle the **olive oil** around the edge of each parmesan egg, then cover the pan with a lid or baking sheet. Cook the eggs for 1 minute or so, until the yolks are set and the whites are crispy and golden on the edges and undersides.

- Remove the pan from the heat and, using a spatula, lift the eggs onto a plate. Arrange the dressed broccoli alongside and sprinkle with **za'atar**, if using, to serve.

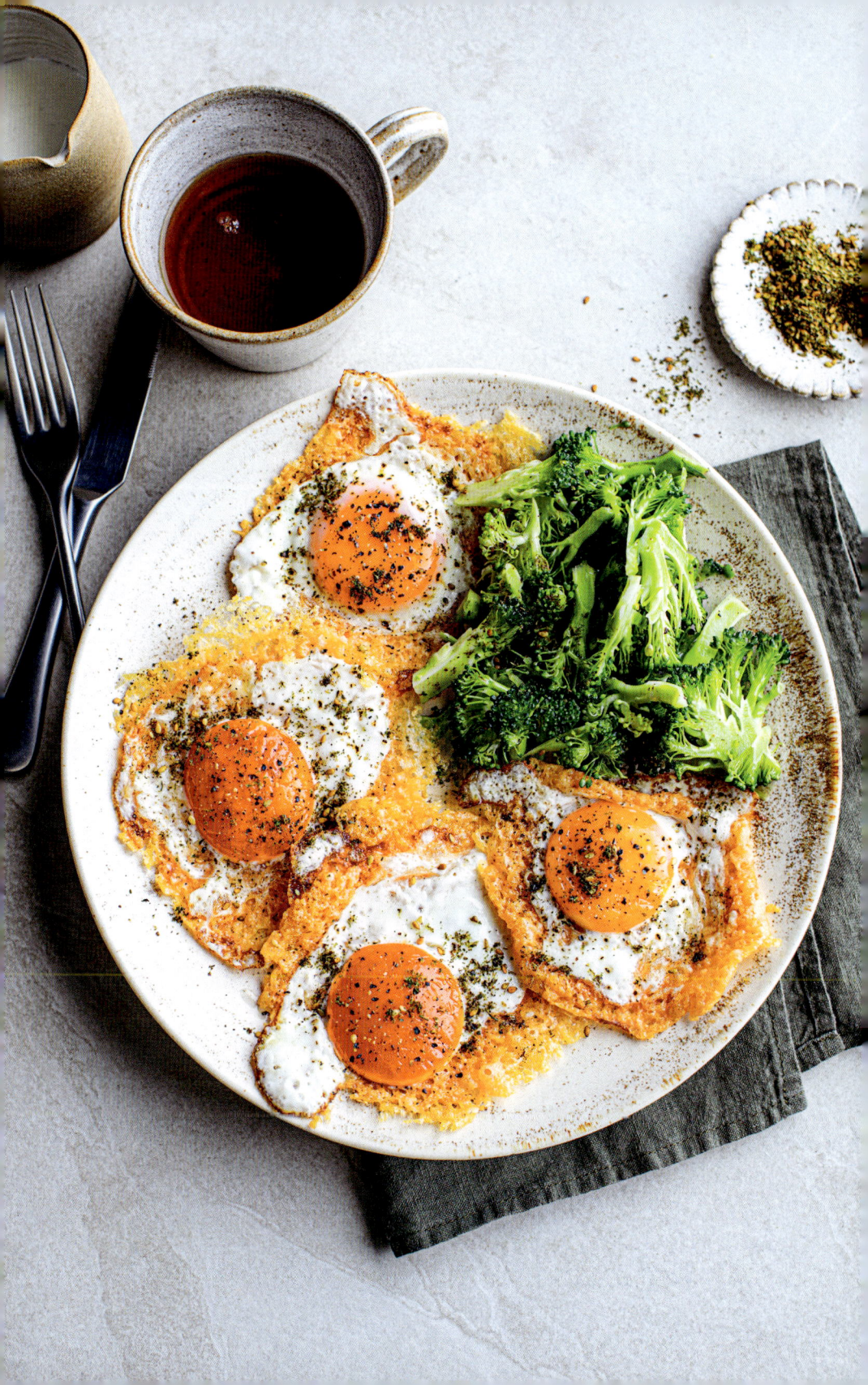

Baked Feta

Ever since my roommate in college showed me how to bake feta, I've never looked back. In this recipe, you can serve the spinach tossed with the other warm vegetables, or keep it on the side as a simple salad. Either way, you're layering in extra folate, vitamin C, and antioxidants. For even more flavor (and a boost of carotenoids), try adding red peppers to the roasting pan with the cherry tomatoes. I love this with some sourdough bread, and—while it can make two portions—I'd often have it all to myself!

SERVES: 2

6 oz (170g) cherry tomatoes
Scant ½ cup (100g) cooked chickpeas from a can or jar, drained and rinsed
1 thyme sprig, stem removed
1 garlic clove, finely sliced (optional)

salt and freshly ground black pepper
7 oz (200g) block of pasteurized feta
3 tbsps olive oil
a handful of baby spinach leaves

OPTIONAL EXTRAS:
finely grated zest of ½ unwaxed lemon
pinch of crushed dried chile flakes

mixed nuts or seeds, toasted, to serve

PER PORTION (WITHOUT OPTIONAL EXTRAS): ✓ 20g protein ✓ 45mg choline

- Heat the oven to 400°F.

- Tip the **cherry tomatoes** into a small roasting pan and add the **chickpeas** and **thyme** and the sliced **garlic**, if using.

- Season lightly with **salt** (the feta is already salty) and more generously with **pepper**. Nestle the **feta** in the middle of the pan among the chickpeas and tomatoes and drizzle with **olive oil**. Sprinkle with the optional extra **lemon zest** and/or **chile flakes**, if using.

- Bake in the middle of the hot oven for 15–20 minutes, until the tomatoes have softened and are just starting to burst and the edges of the feta are golden and crisp.

- Stir in the **baby spinach** and allow it to wilt in the heat of the vegetables, then serve, sprinkled with toasted **nuts or seeds**, if you wish.

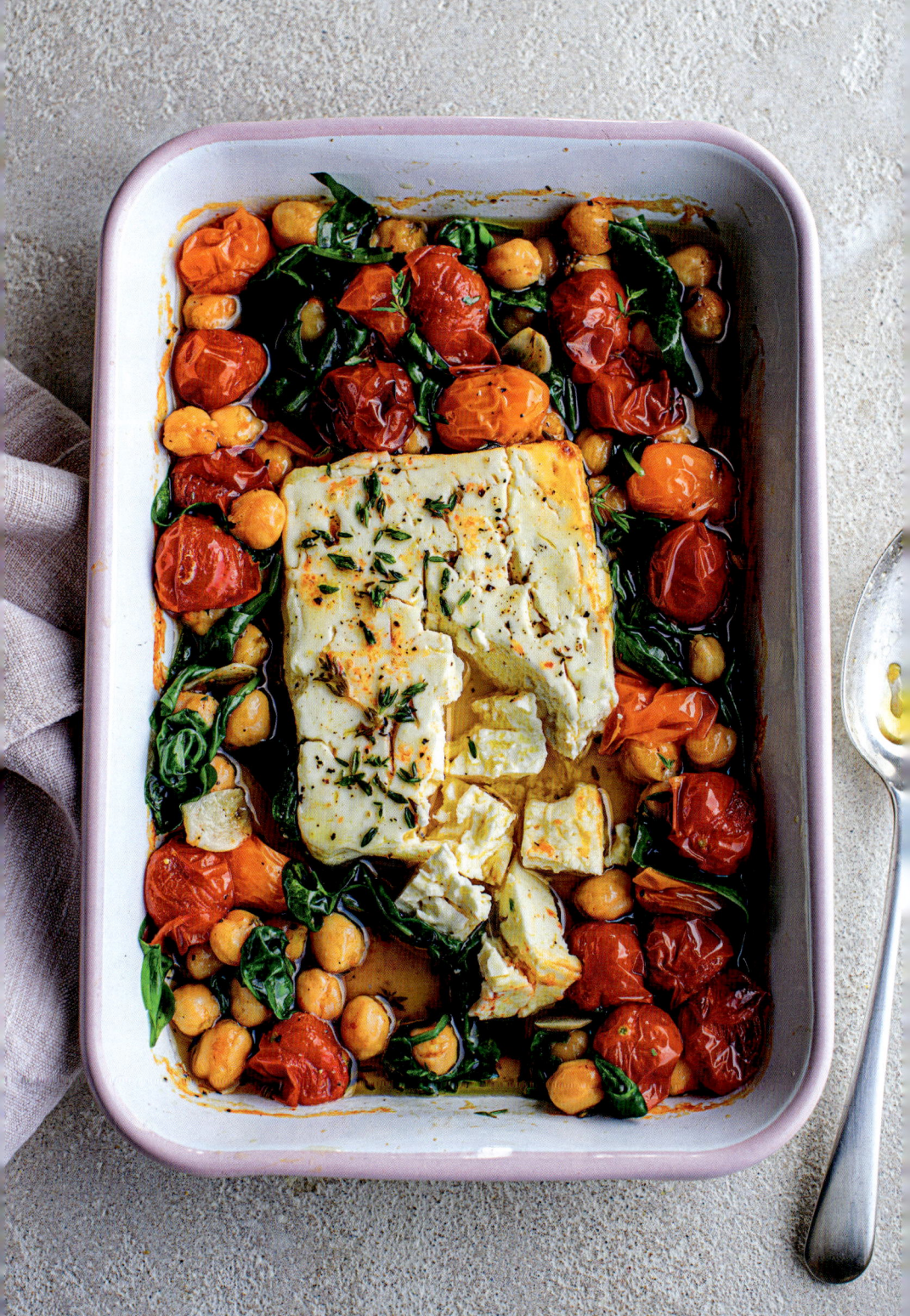

MAIN DISHES

Lima Beans with Greens and Sardines

This dish is everything you need in pregnancy food: simple, hearty, and bursting with protein, choline, and a huge hit of DHA thanks to the sardines.

SERVES: 1

- 2 tbsps olive oil
- 1 garlic clove, crushed to a paste
- 1 x 15-oz (425g) can of lima beans (butter beans), drained
- a handful of baby spinach
- 7 oz (200g) chard or kale, roughly chopped
- juice of ½ lemon
- salt and freshly ground black pepper
- 1 x 4.4-oz (125g) tin of sardines in olive oil, drained

PER PORTION (THE WHOLE RECIPE): ✓ 40g protein ✓ 287mg choline ✓ 1,950mg DHA

- Heat the **olive oil** in a large frying pan over medium heat. Add the **garlic** and cook for 30 seconds, until aromatic, but do not brown. Add the **lima beans** and cook for 1–2 minutes to warm through.

- Add the **spinach** and **chard or kale** and a splash of water and cook, stirring gently, until the leaves have just wilted.

- Slide the pan off the heat, add the **lemon juice**, and season well with **salt** and **pepper**. Tip the beans and greens into a serving dish, flake the sardines on top, and serve.

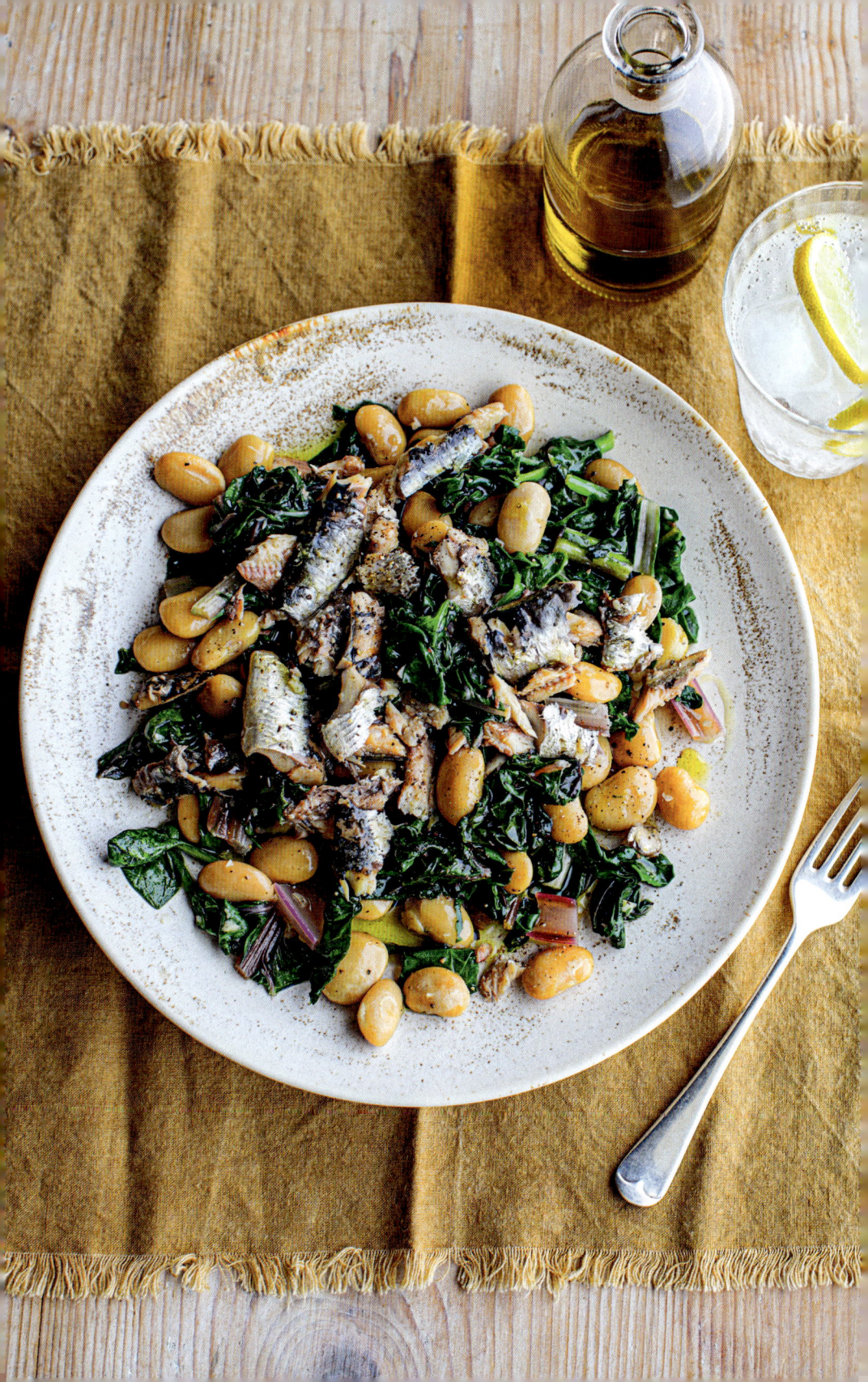

Smash Parmesan Patties

This was one of my pregnancy staples—and yes, I really mean two patties, not just one. Meat is a direct source of the building blocks your baby needs. So, if you can manage it, go for two. And because I can never resist, I always finish my patties with a snowfall of parmesan on top. Serve them with some beans or salad, or riff on the seasonings to keep it interesting: a splash of Worcestershire sauce, a little Tabasco, some chopped pickles or shallots . . . whatever makes it delicious for you.

SERVES: 1

7 oz (200g) good-quality ground beef
1 garlic clove, crushed to a paste
1 tbsp Dijon mustard
1 thyme sprig, stem removed
½ tsp paprika (smoked or sweet, both work)
salt and freshly ground black pepper
1 tbsp olive oil
2 tbsps freshly grated parmesan, to serve

PER PORTION (THE WHOLE RECIPE): ✓ 58g protein ✓ 160mg choline

- In a medium bowl, combine the **ground beef** with the **garlic, Dijon mustard, thyme,** and **paprika** and sprinkle generously with **salt** and **pepper**. Mix well to combine and shape the mixture into two balls. Cover and chill for 20 minutes, or until ready to cook.

- Heat the **olive oil** in a large frying pan over high heat. Using your hands, flatten the meat balls into patties and place them into the hot pan. Using a spatula, flatten each patty to a thickness of about ½ inch (1cm) and cook for about 3 minutes on each side, until cooked through and browned.

- Transfer the patties to a plate and serve topped with a mound of freshly grated **parmesan** on top and your chosen greens alongside.

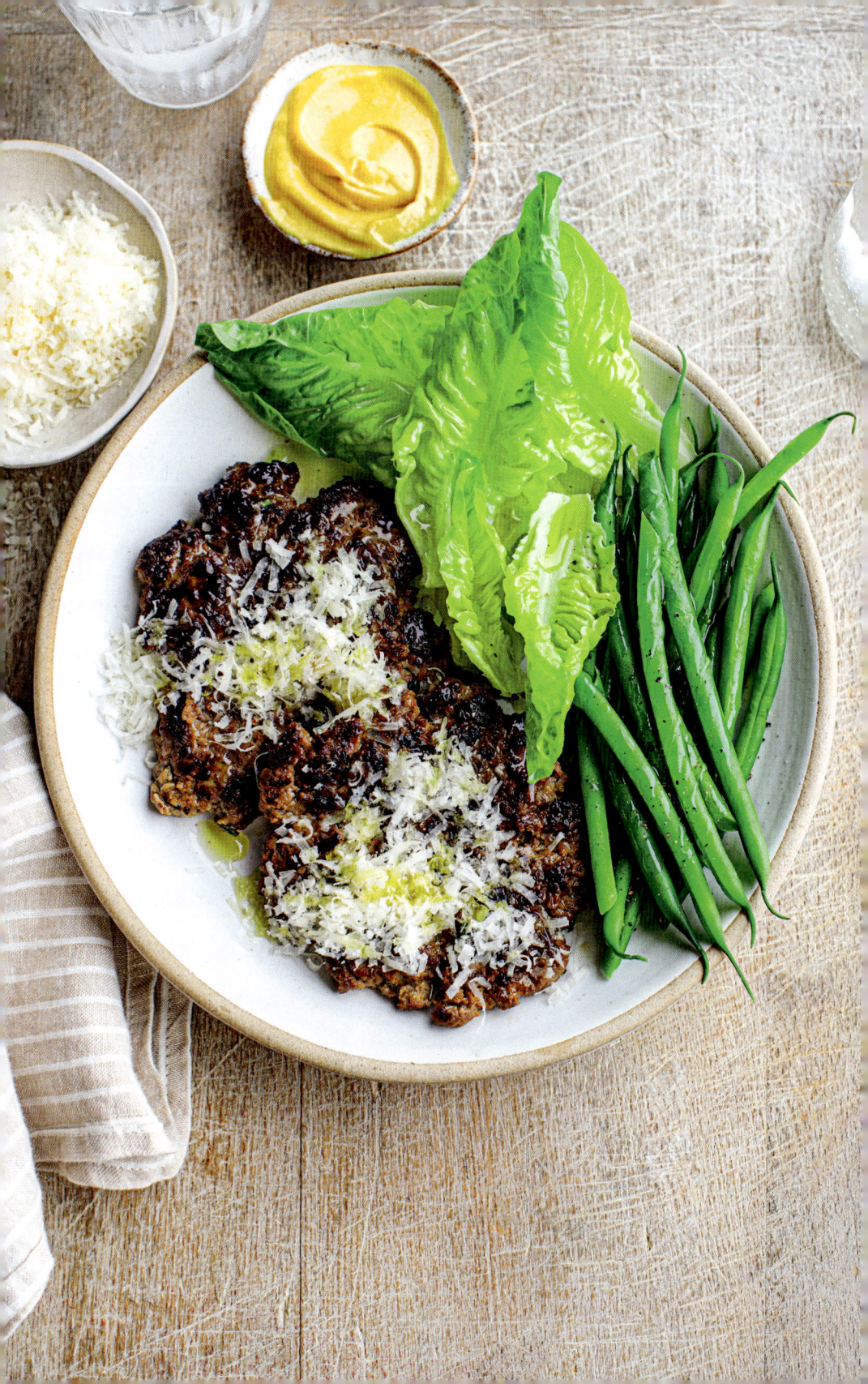

Salmon and Feta Fishcakes

These salmon and feta fishcakes check every box. They're also versatile: have one straight from the pan as a snack, or serve four with a salad for a full meal. The dill, lemon zest, and capers keep things fresh and zippy, while the feta adds a salty kick. Reheat them either in the microwave or wrapped in foil and popped into the oven at 350°F for 10 minutes.

MAKES: 12 FISHCAKES/3 PORTIONS

14 oz (400g) skinless salmon fillet
4 oz (115g) pasteurized feta, crumbled
1 rounded tbsp drained capers
finely grated zest of ½ unwaxed lemon
2 tbsps chopped dill
1 egg, beaten
salt and freshly ground black pepper
2–3 tbsps olive oil
2 tbsps all-purpose flour
a spoonful of tzatziki (store-bought), to serve
lemon wedges, to serve

PER PORTION (4 FISHCAKES/ONE THIRD OF THE RECIPE): ✓ 37g protein
✓ 185mg choline ✓ 1,950 mg DHA (if you use free-range pasture-raised eggs)

• Cut the **salmon** into dice and tip into a food processor. Pulse until the salmon is chopped into small pieces, then tip it into a bowl and add the **feta**.

• Roughly chop the **capers**, add them to the salmon with the **lemon zest**, **dill**, and **egg**, and sprinkle with **salt** and **pepper**. Mix to thoroughly combine, then shape the mixture into 12 equal size patties.

• Heat the **olive oil** in a large frying pan over medium heat. Dust the fishcakes in the **flour** to coat and then, in batches, fry the fishcakes for about 2 minutes on one side, then flip and cook on the other side, until golden all over and thoroughly cooked through.

• Serve hot with a good dollop of **tzatziki** and **lemon wedges** for squeezing over the top.

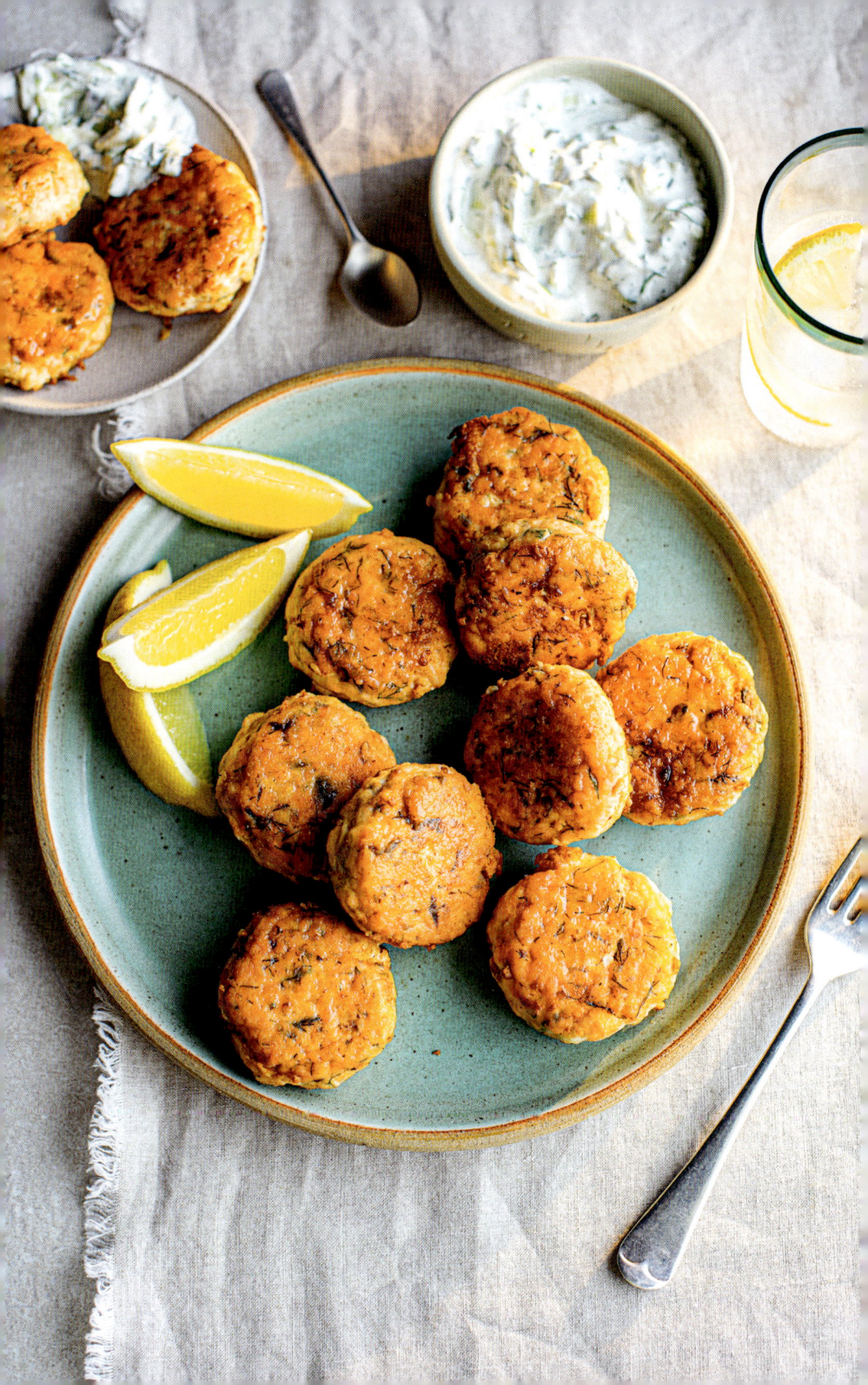

Chicken Caesar

This salad is my riff on a chicken Caesar, with kale stepping in for the lettuce (you can also use Romaine) and a creamy avocado-cashew dressing. It's not just delicious, it's a building-block bomb.

SERVES: 2

2 boneless skinless chicken breasts
5–7 oz (140–200g) kale leaves
2 tbsps pumpkin seeds, toasted

FOR THE DRESSING:

1 small ripe avocado (or ½ large avocado)
⅓ cup (50g) unsalted cashews
1 garlic clove
2 tbsps roughly chopped flat-leaf parsley
8 tbsps (120ml) extra-virgin olive oil
juice of 1 small lemon
¼ cup (25g) freshly grated parmesan, plus extra (shaved or grated) to serve
salt and freshly ground black pepper

PER PORTION (HALF THE RECIPE): ✓ 54g protein ✓ 180mg choline

- First, make the dressing. Cut the **avocado** flesh into chunks and tip them into a high-speed blender. Add the **cashews, garlic, flat-leaf parsley**, 7 tablespoons (100ml) of the **extra-virgin olive oil**, and the **lemon juice**. Add the **parmesan** and 3 tablespoons of cold water and season well with **salt** and **pepper**. Blend until the dressing is smooth, and set aside.

- Place the **chicken breasts** between two sheets of plastic wrap or parchment paper and, using a rolling pin or the bottom of a heavy saucepan or frying pan, bash the chicken to slightly flatten each breast to a thickness of around ½ inch (1cm).

- Heat the remaining 1 tablespoon oil in a frying pan over medium-high heat. Add the chicken breasts and cook for about 3 minutes on each side, until golden brown and cooked through. Remove them from the pan and let cool.

- Tear the **kale** into bite-size pieces and tip them into a large bowl. Add two-thirds of the dressing and toss the leaves to coat.

- Divide the dressed kale between two serving plates. Slice the chicken breasts and place equal amounts on top of the kale, drizzle with more dressing, scatter the **pumpkin seeds**, and sprinkle with more parmesan to serve.

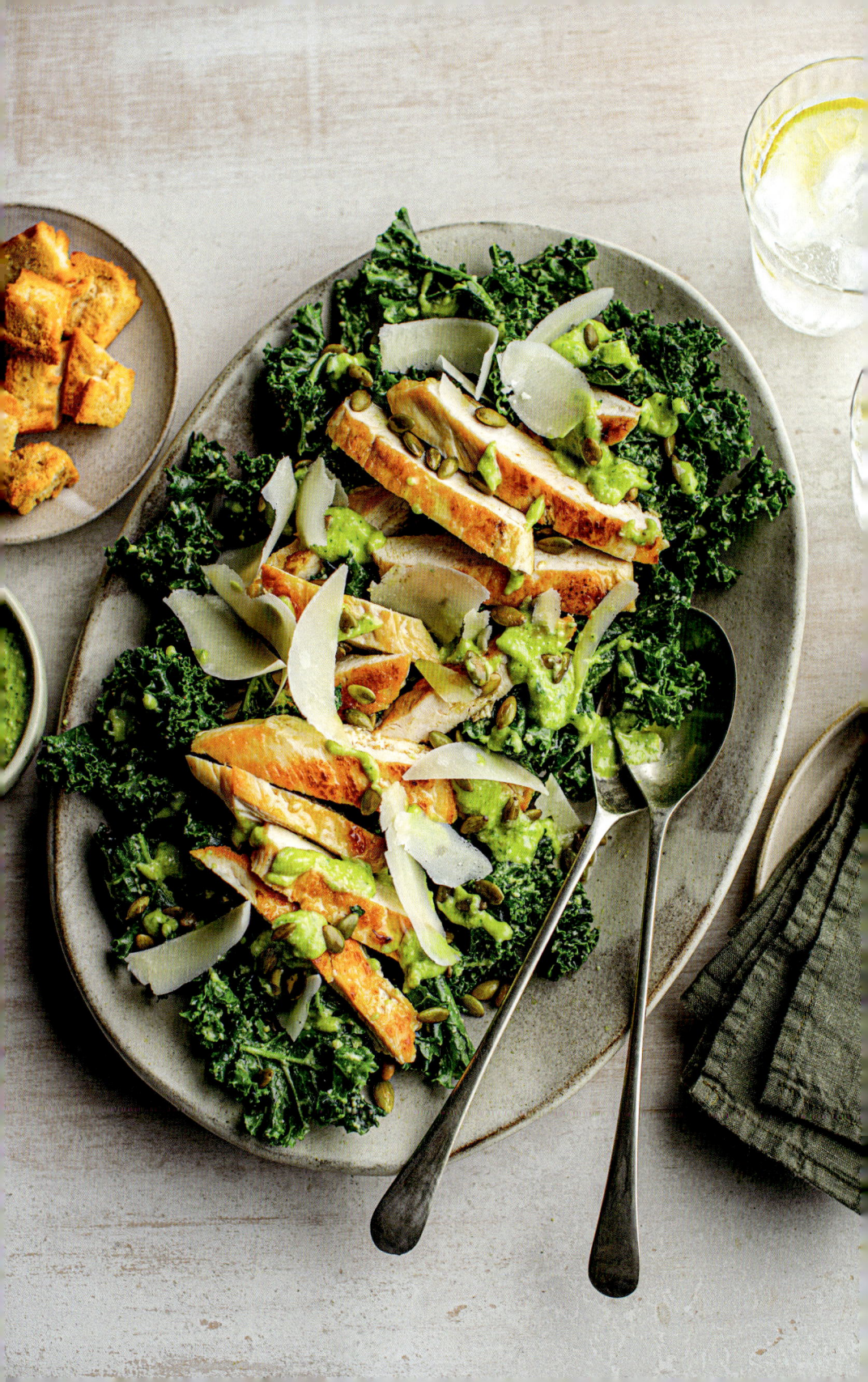

Pistachio Pesto Steak Night

Steak night, Jessie edition. The queen of this dish is definitely the pistachio pesto. Sure, you could grab a jar of store-bought pesto, but making your own turns a simple steak into something special—and adds extra protein, choline, and healthy fats in the process. The pesto in this recipe yields enough for two servings and will keep happily in the fridge for three to four days, ready to upgrade your next meal.

SERVES: 1 (WITH 1 PORTION OF LEFTOVER PESTO)

1 x 7 oz (200g) sirloin steak
4 oz (115g) cherry tomatoes, halved

a handful of arugula, watercress, or baby spinach leaves

FOR THE PISTACHIO PESTO:
½ cup (50g) shelled unsalted pistachios
½ small bunch of flat-leaf parsley
½ small bunch of basil
1 garlic clove

3 tbsps grated parmesan, plus extra shavings to serve
5 tbsps (75ml) extra-virgin olive oil
salt and freshly ground black pepper
juice of ½ lemon, optional, to taste

PER PORTION: ✓ 60g protein ✓ 180mg choline

- Start by making the pistachio pesto. Tip the **pistachios, flat-leaf parsley, basil,** and **garlic** into a mini food processor and blend until finely chopped.

- Add the **parmesan** and 4 tablespoons (60ml) of the **extra-virgin olive oil,** season with **salt** and **pepper,** and pulse until combined. Add **lemon juice** to taste, if you like.

- Heat the remaining 1 tablespoon olive oil in a frying pan over high heat. Sprinkle the **steak** with salt and pepper and cook for about 4 minutes on each side, until nicely charred all over and cooked through. Remove the steak from the pan and set it aside to rest for 5 minutes.

- Tip the **cherry tomatoes** into the hot pan and quickly cook them over high heat for 30–60 seconds to soften them slightly.

- Arrange the **salad leaves** on a plate and scatter the tomatoes. Slice the steak into ½-inch (1cm)-thick slices and arrange it on top of the leaves. Drizzle the pesto and shave a little parmesan over the top to serve.

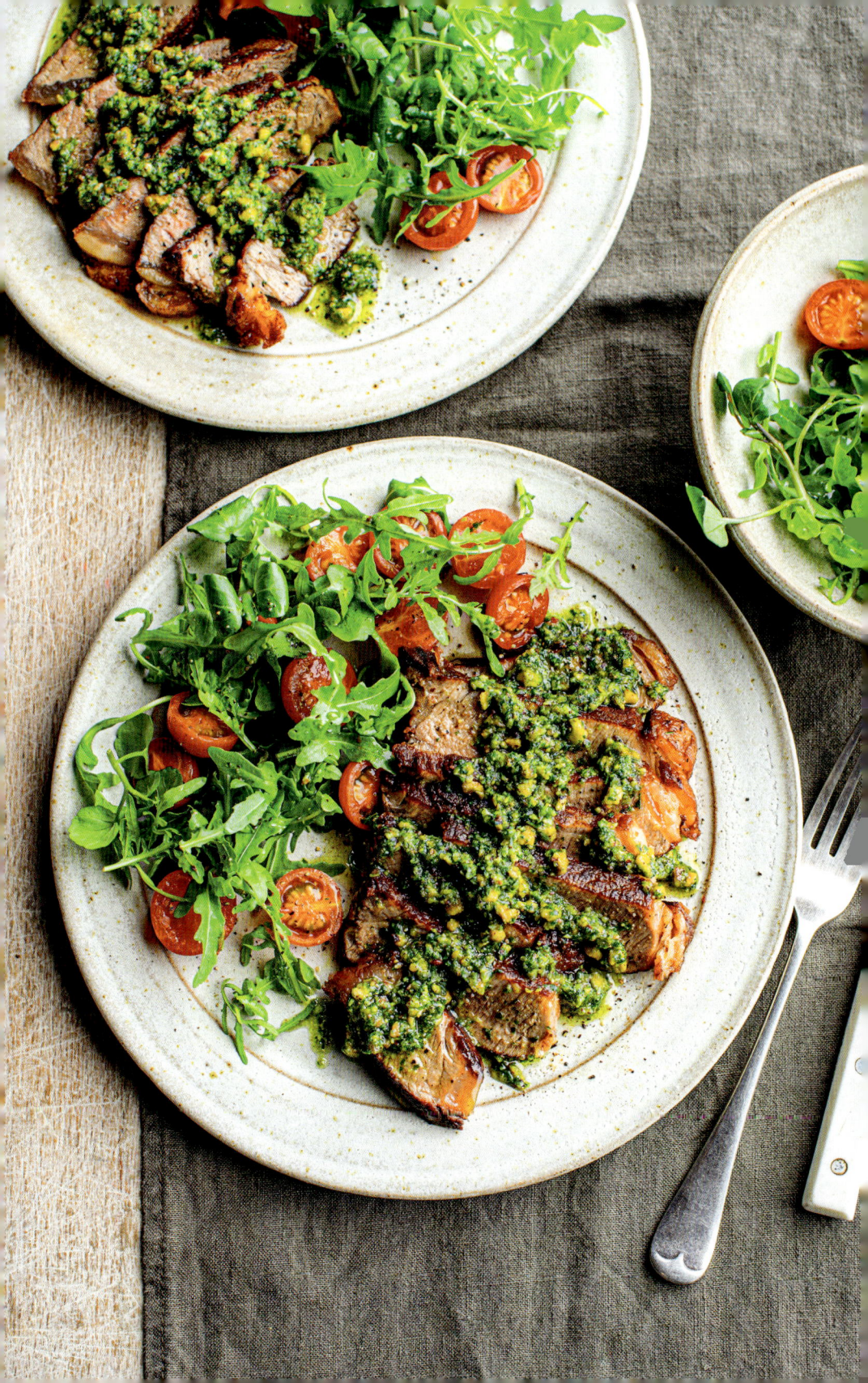

The Baby Salad

Do you remember, in Chapter 5, how I explained that the dark colors in fruit and vegetables are a signal of powerful phytonutrients? This baby salad is a perfect example.

SERVES: 2

2 beets, rinsed but not peeled
1 red bell pepper, quartered and seeded
6 tbsps (90ml) extra-virgin olive oil
2 tbsps roasted tahini
juice of ½ lemon
1 garlic clove, crushed to a paste

salt and freshly ground black pepper
4 oz (115g) baby spinach
¾ cup (175g) cooked chickpeas from a can or jar, drained and rinsed
1 tsp za'atar (optional)
2–3 tbsps Greek yogurt, to serve

PROTEIN ADD-INS
3 hard-boiled eggs, or 1 cooked chicken breast, or 5 oz (140g) tofu

PER PORTION + 3 EGGS: ✓ 32g protein ✓ 444mg choline ✓ 90mg DHA
+ 1 CHICKEN BREAST: ✓ 56g protein ✓ 182mg choline
+ 150G FIRM TOFU: ✓ 23g protein ✓ 111mg choline

- Start by roasting the **beets** and **bell pepper**. Heat the oven to 350°F and line a small roasting pan with parchment paper. Cut each beet into quarters or sixths, depending on size, and tip the wedges into the prepared pan. Drizzle with 1 tablespoon of the **extra-virgin olive oil** and season well with **salt** and **pepper**. Roast the beets for about 15 minutes, until they are starting to soften.

- Add the quartered red bell pepper to the roasting pan, drizzle with another 1 tablespoon of the olive oil, and return the pan to the oven for 15 minutes, until all the vegetables are tender and starting to char at the edges.

- Meanwhile, prepare the dressing. In a bowl, combine the **tahini, lemon juice,** and **garlic**. Add the remaining 4 tablespoons (60ml) of olive oil and season with salt and pepper. Whisk to combine and add a little cold water, if the dressing is a little thick.

- Divide the **spinach** between two plates and top each portion with half of the **chickpeas** and roasted veggies. Season with **za'atar**, if using, and drizzle with the dressing.

- Serve with a dollop of **Greek yogurt** on the side and whichever protein option you prefer.

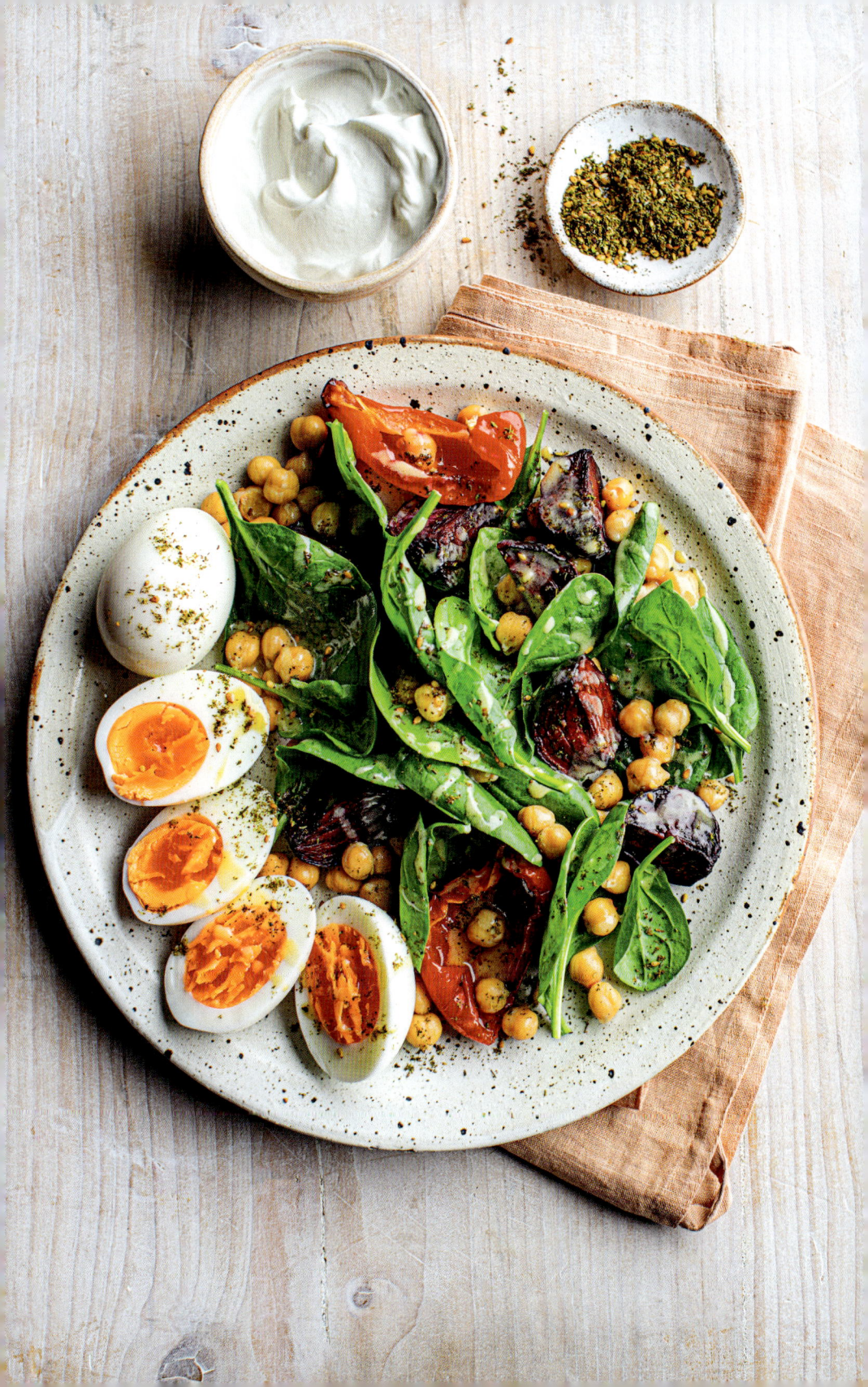

SNACKS

My Absolute Favorite Snack

Allow me to start this section with the snack I ate almost every day in my second and third trimesters—my pregnancy obsession. It was the perfect, tasty way get a whopping dose of protein in one go, plus a nice boost of choline and a burst of colorful fruit. And on mornings when I didn't feel like eggs, it doubled as the perfect breakfast. I used a grass-fed whey isolate protein powder (see my recommendations here: glucosegoddess.com/pages/best-protein-powders). And trust me on the sea-salt flakes—they bring it all together.

SERVES: 1

Scant 1 cup (250g) Icelandic-style yogurt (such as Skyr)
a portion of high-quality protein powder to yield 20g of protein
1 tbsp nut butter
a small handful of whole, skin-on (not blanched) nuts, such as pecans, almonds, or hazelnuts
a handful of fruit, such as berries, kiwi, banana, peaches, or nectarines
seeds and juice from ½ passion fruit
a pinch of sea-salt flakes

PER PORTION (THE WHOLE RECIPE): ✓ 58g protein ✓ 115mg choline

- Mix the **yogurt** and **protein powder** in a serving bowl until smooth and thoroughly combined (this may take a minute). Spoon the **nut butter** on top.

- Roughly chop the **nuts** and add them to the bowl, sprinkling them over the yogurt.

- Prepare the **fruit** of your choice—cut larger berries into halves or quarters; peel and slice banana and kiwi; cut peaches and nectarines into bite-size slices.

- Arrange the fruit on top of the nuts and yogurt, spoon the **passion fruit** seeds and juice on top, and add a light sprinkle of **sea-salt flakes** to finish. Enjoy.

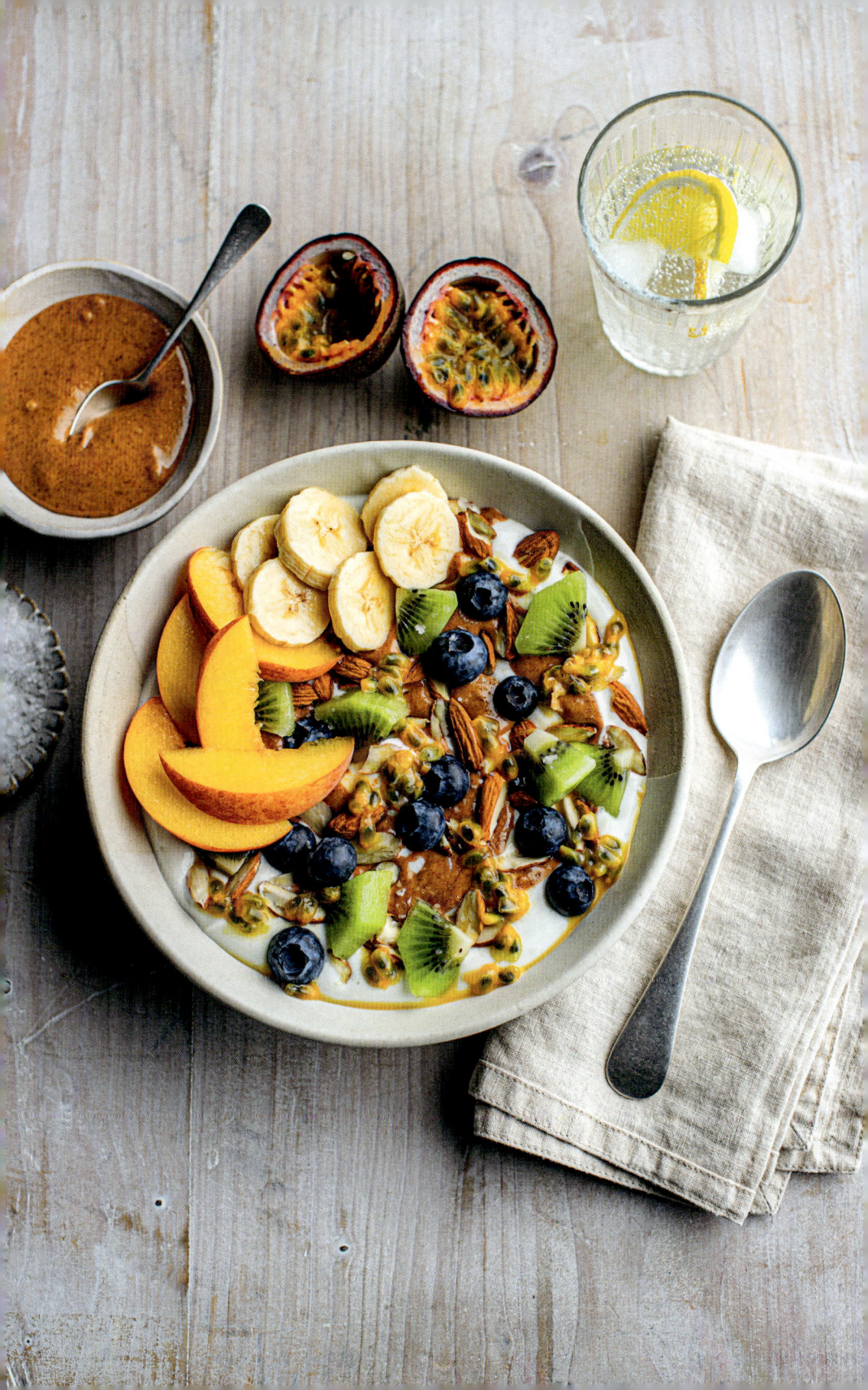

Cauliflower with Chickpeas

Chickpeas and cauliflower are some of the best choline-rich foods in the plant kingdom, so I had them as my main plant foods during pregnancy. If you eat fish, add a side of tinned salmon and you'll bring this bowl up to around 32g of protein and 200mg of choline per serving—*and* turn its negligible DHA into a fabulous 500mg. To pump this salad up, add some warmed mixed grains or lentils—precooked grains in a pouch are a brilliant pantry standby.

SERVES: 2

½ cauliflower (including leaves)
4 tbsps (60ml) extra-virgin olive oil
1 tsp cumin seeds
½ tsp chile flakes or smoked paprika
salt and freshly ground black pepper

scant 1 cup (200g) cooked chickpeas from a can or jar, drained and rinsed
scant 1 cup (200g) hummus (made with roasted tahini)
2 tbsps pomegranate seeds

PER PORTION: ✓ 18g protein ✓ 140mg choline

- Heat the oven to 400°F.

- Cut the **cauliflower** into bite-size florets (reserve the leaves). Tip the pieces into a small roasting pan, drizzle with 2 tablespoons of the **extra-virgin olive oil**, sprinkle with the **cumin seeds** and **chile flakes** or **smoked paprika**, and season with **salt** and **pepper**. Roast the cauliflower for about 12 minutes, until it is tender and starting to char at the edges.

- Add the cauliflower leaves and **chickpeas** to the pan, shake the pan to coat them in the oil, and roast for 5–6 minutes, or until the leaves are starting to brown and crisp.

- Spoon the **hummus** equally over two serving plates and make a well in the middle of each portion. Arrange the cauliflower florets, leaves, and chickpeas on top, scatter the **pomegranate seeds**, and drizzle with the remaining 2 tablespoons of olive oil to serve.

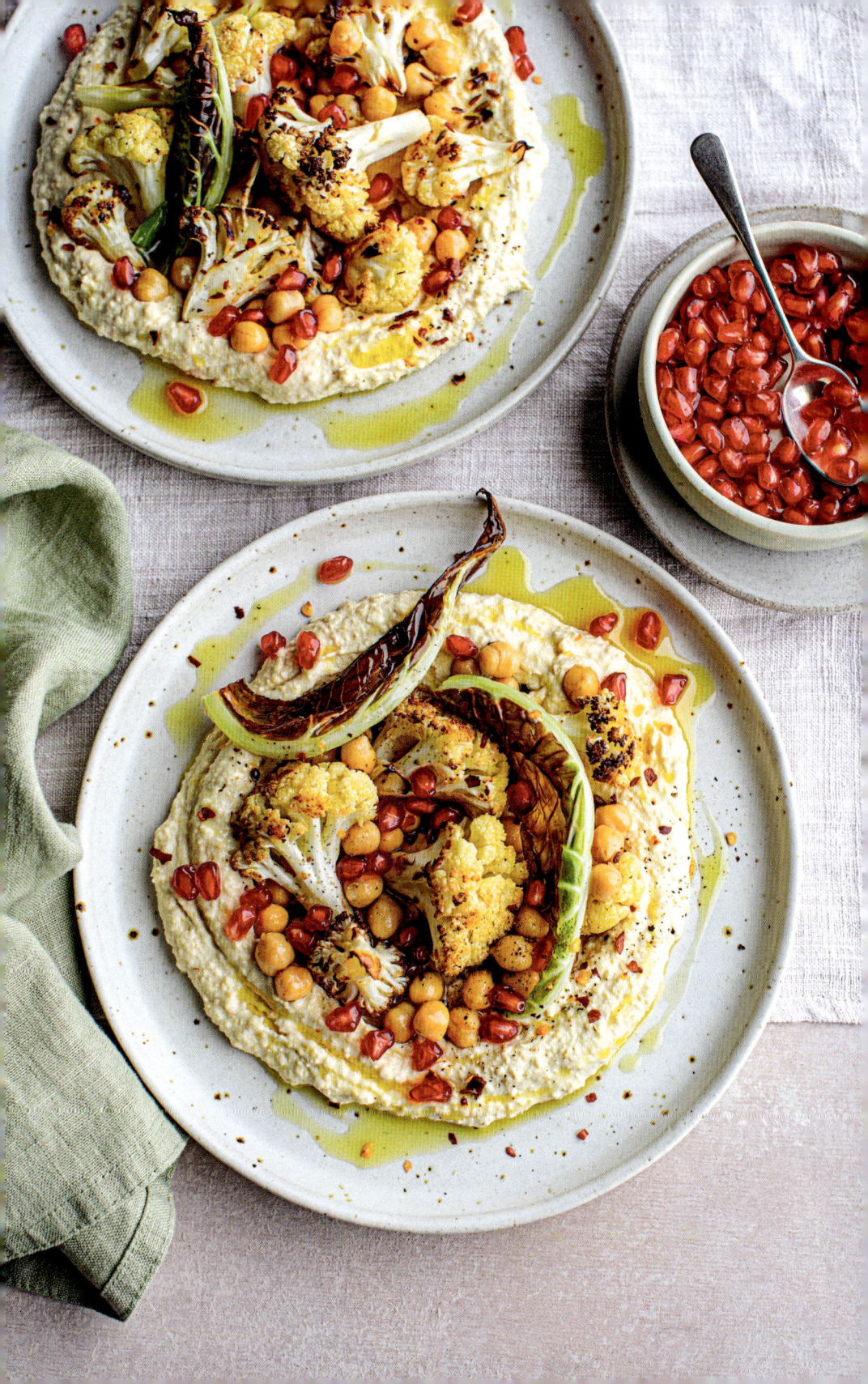

Crispy Chickpeas

These make the perfect snack, but you can also add them to salads or use them as a topper for soups. Try switching the spices around to suit your taste. Powdered wasabi is a good option for extra heat, za'atar is a wonderful warming spice blend, and if all else fails medium-heat curry powder is always tasty.

MAKES: 3 PORTIONS

1 x 15-oz (425g) can of chickpeas
1 tsp ground cumin
½ tsp cayenne
1 tsp smoked paprika
½ tsp garlic granules
1–2 tbsp olive oil
salt and freshly ground black pepper

PER PORTION (ONE THIRD OF THE RECIPE): ✓ 7g protein ✓ 15mg choline

- Heat the oven to 400°F and line a baking sheet with parchment paper and a plate with paper towels.

- Drain and rinse the **chickpeas** and tip them onto the plate lined with paper towels to dry slightly.

- In a medium bowl, combine the **ground cumin, cayenne, smoked paprika,** and **garlic granules**. Add the chickpeas and 1 tablespoon of the **olive oil** and season well with **salt** and **pepper**. Mix well to coat the chickpeas in the spices, adding the remaining 1 tablespoon of the olive oil if needed for an even coating, then tip them into the lined baking sheet, shimmying them into an even layer.

- Roast the chickpeas for 30–35 minutes, until crispy, shaking the baking sheet from time to time so that they cook evenly. Let cool before serving. You can store them in an airtight container in the fridge for up to 3 days.

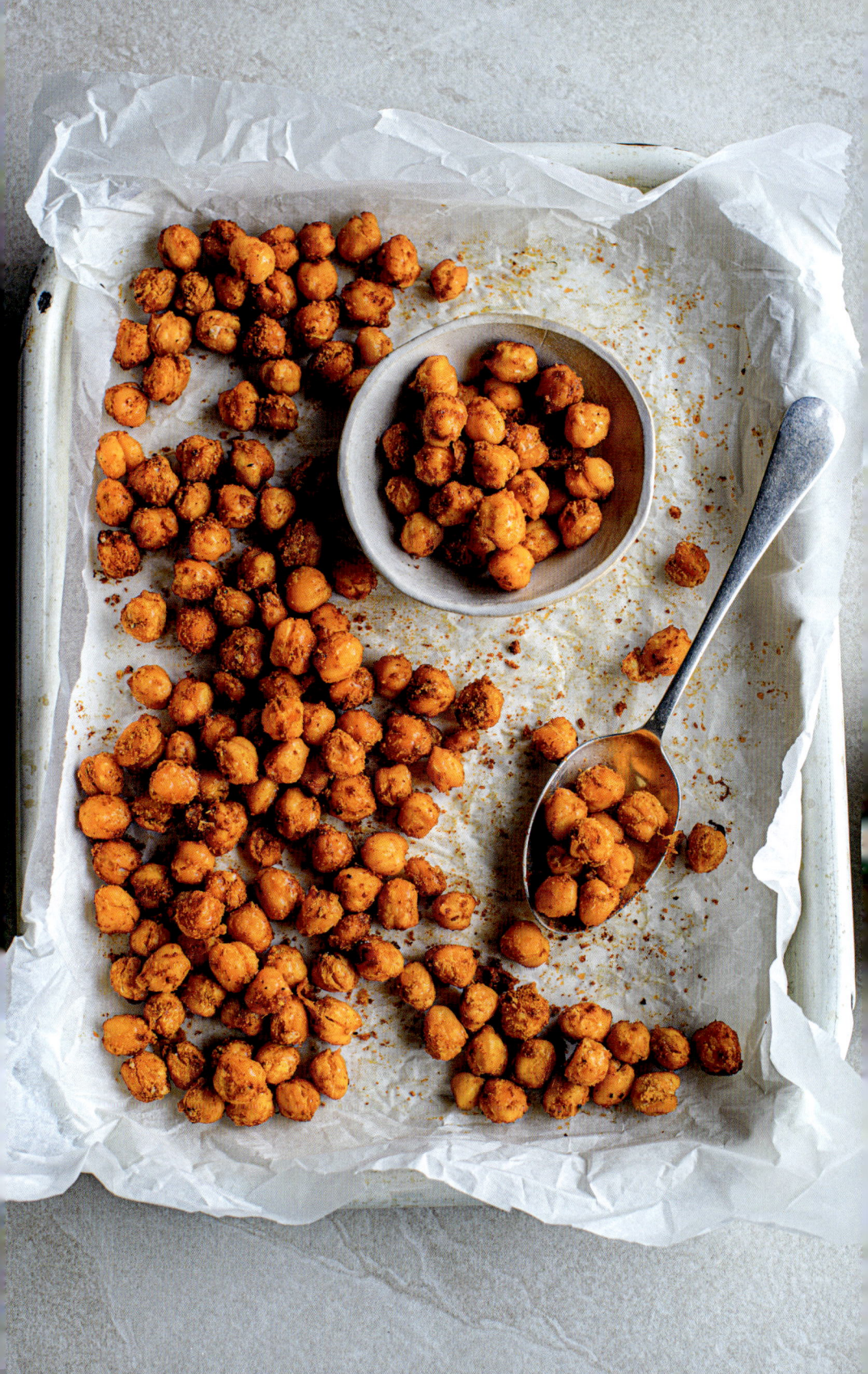

Nori and Seed Crackers

In Chapter 4, I told you about nori sheets as a great source of iodine. This recipe makes about 24 crackers, but just half the batch will get you 100mcg out of your daily 250mcg iodine goal, while also adding a good dose of plant-based protein from the seeds and a helpful boost of choline.

MAKES: 2 PORTIONS (EACH OF ABOUT 12 CRACKERS)

1¼ cups (150g) mixed seeds (pumpkin, sunflower, sesame, flax, and hemp)
2 tbsps chia seeds
⅓ cup (50g) ground flaxseed

¼ cup (25g) grated parmesan
2 sheets of nori
salt and freshly ground black pepper

PER PORTION (HALF THE RECIPE): ✓ 34g protein ✓ 65mg choline ✓ 100mcg iodine

- Heat the oven to 275°F and line one large or two medium baking sheets with parchment paper.

- Tip the **mixed seeds** into a medium bowl. Add the **chia seeds, ground flaxseed**, and **parmesan**.

- Cut the **nori sheets** into rough pieces. Tip them into a mini food processor and pulse until the nori is chopped into about ¼ inch (6mm) pieces. Add this to the seed mixture and season well with **salt** and **pepper**.

- Add ⅔ cup (160ml) of cold water and mix well to combine until the mixture clumps. A small spoonful at a time, add more water, if needed, to bring it together.

- Using an offset spatula, spread the mixture thinly and evenly onto the prepared baking sheets—it should be 1/16–⅛ inch (2–3mm) thick. Bake for about 50 minutes, turning the sheets around halfway through baking, until the cracker is evenly dry and crisp. Flip the cracker over so that the underside is now uppermost and return it to the oven for 20 minutes to dry out.

- Allow the cracker to cool on the baking sheet, then break it into individual, cracker-size pieces (you should get about 24 evenly sized pieces). Serve with cream cheese, if you like. Store in airtight food containers for up to 3 days.

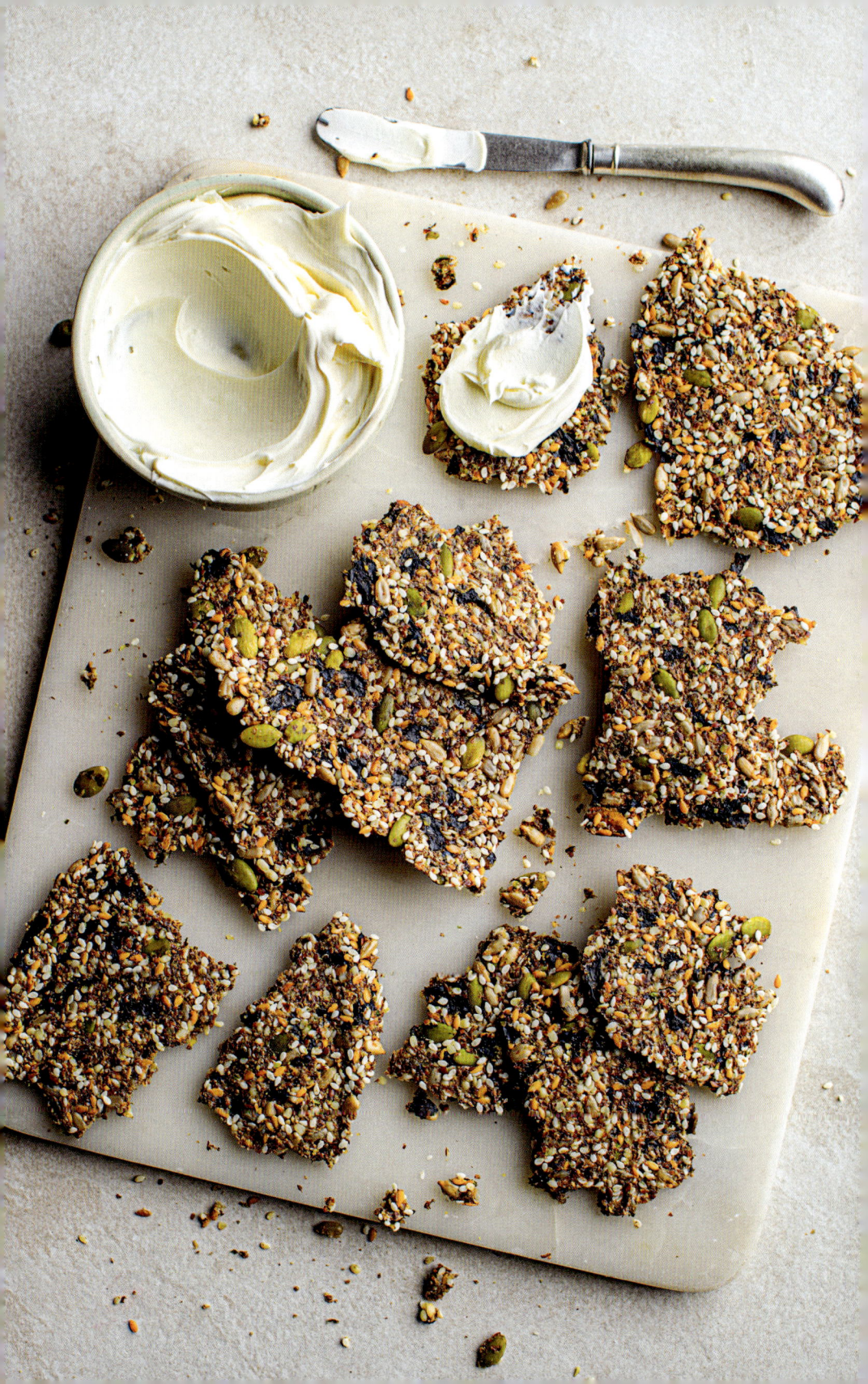

Peach and Mozzarella Salad

When I learned how much protein was in mozzarella, I was very happy. There are 21g in a standard mozzarella ball—the same as in three eggs! Mozzarella is generally pasteurized, so it's safe to eat during pregnancy. It is also—like all dairy products—a source of iodine. Not bad, right?

SERVES: 1

a handful of arugula leaves
1 ripe peach
a handful of mixed tomatoes
1 avocado or 1 baby cucumber
4 oz (115g) ball of pasteurized mozzarella, drained

2 basil sprigs, stems removed
1–2 tbsps extra-virgin olive oil
2 tsps white wine vinegar or apple cider vinegar
salt and freshly ground black pepper

PER PORTION (THE WHOLE RECIPE): ✓ 25g protein ✓ 54mg choline ✓ 60mcg iodine

- Scatter the **arugula** leaves onto a plate. Cut the **peach** flesh into wedges, slice the **tomatoes** into bite-size pieces, slice the **avocado or cucumber,** and arrange these on top.

- Tear the **mozzarella** into bite-size pieces and nestle the pieces among the peaches. Roughly tear the **basil** leaves and scatter them over the top.

- Drizzle with the **extra-virgin olive oil** (more or less, according to taste) and **white wine vinegar or apple cider vinegar.** Season with **salt** and **pepper** and serve.

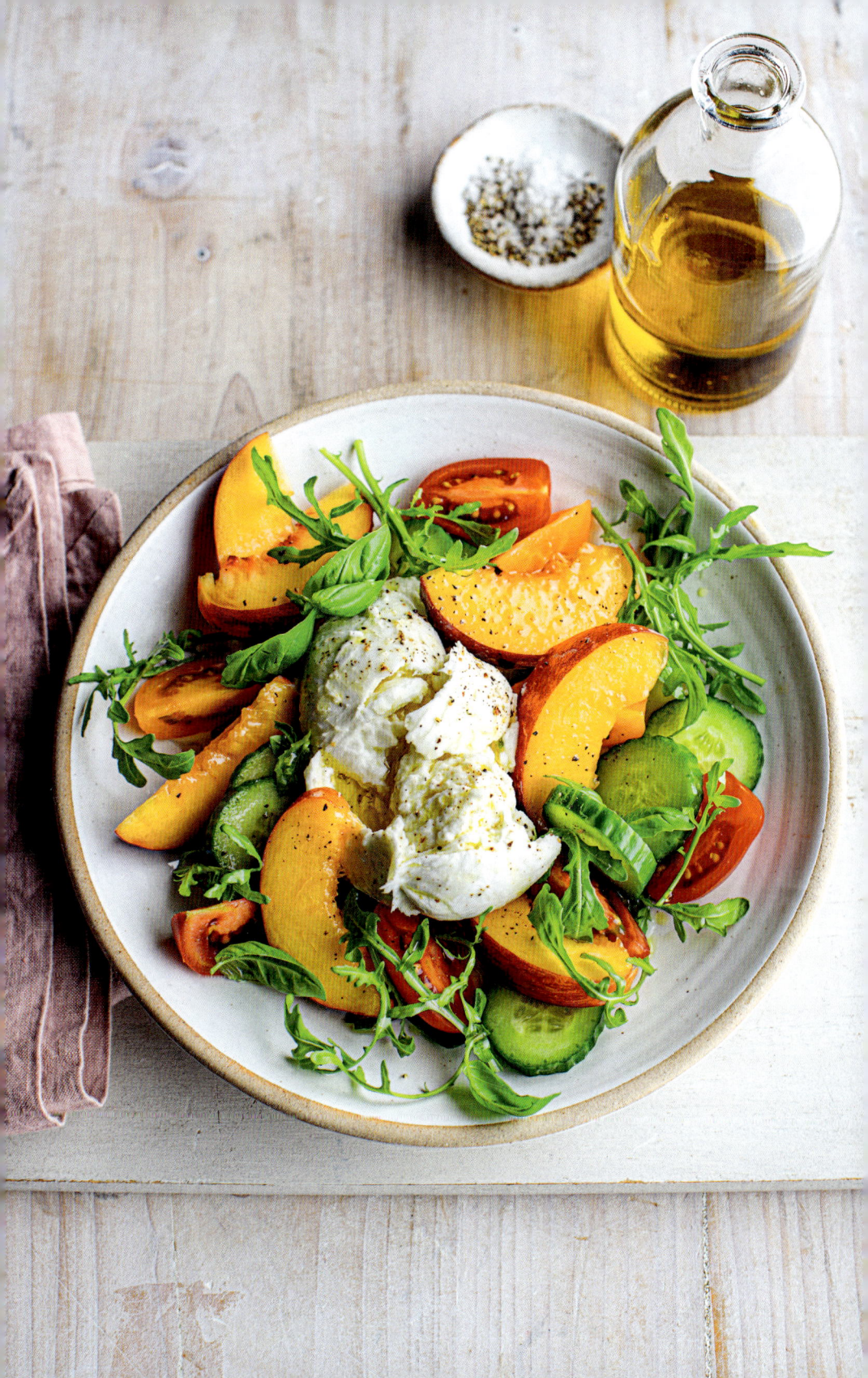

Savory Baked Oat Bars

These delicious savory squares are an ideal snack to have in the fridge, in your handbag for when you are out, or tucked into a lunchbox for a day at work. They contain starch in the rolled oats, but because they are paired with so much fiber and protein, they won't spike your glucose levels. By the way, you can use whichever lentils you prefer. Try adding 2 tablespoons of chopped soft herbs to the mixture, such as flat-leaf parsley, chives, or cilantro, or even add a little spice, such as cumin or a pinch of chile, or a good spoonful of whole grain mustard, if you like.

MAKES: 16 SQUARES

1⅓ cups (125g) rolled oats
1¾ cups (200g) coarsely grated carrot (from about 2 carrots; no need to peel)
⅔ cup (75g) mixed seeds (sunflower, pumpkin, flax, hemp, sesame), plus extra for sprinkling

1⅓ cups (100g) cooked lentils (either green, Le Puy, or black lentils)
1 cup (125g) grated cheddar
2 large eggs, lightly beaten
¼ cup (50g) unsalted butter, melted
salt and freshly ground black pepper

PER SQUARE: ✓ 6g protein ✓ 30mg choline

- Heat the oven to 350°F and line an 8-inch (20cm) square baking pan with parchment paper.

- In a large bowl, combine the **oats, carrot, mixed seeds,** and **cooked lentils**. Add the grated **cheddar** and mix to combine.

- In a small bowl, mix together the **eggs** and melted **butter** and sprinkle generously with **salt** and **pepper**. Add this to the oat mixture and mix well to thoroughly combine.

- Tip into the prepared baking pan and spread level with the back of a spoon. Scatter with **sesame seeds** and bake for about 35 minutes, until golden brown.

- Let cool and then cut into squares to serve.

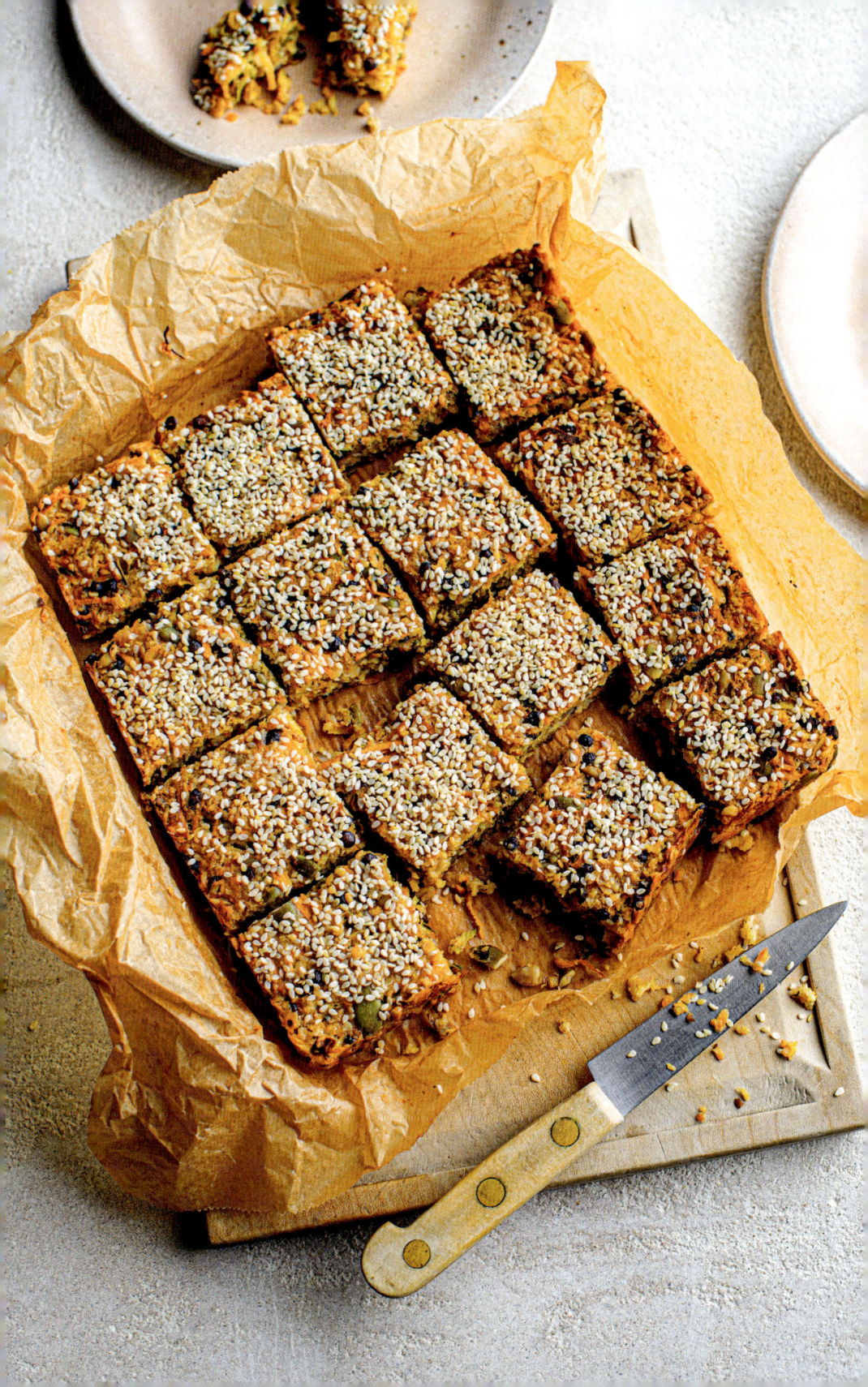

Shiitake Broth with Miso and Cavolo Nero

This miso soup hits the spot when you're craving something salty and comforting. I would often break up a nori sheet in there at the end for a boost of 100mcg iodine. Switch up the green veggies depending on your preference—broccolini or Brussels sprouts are good subs for cavolo nero. You can also add a little grated fresh ginger, sliced red chile, and crushed garlic to the mushrooms for an extra pop of flavor. This recipe makes enough for two portions—one to eat now and one for another day.

SERVES: 2

- 5 oz (140g) shiitake mushrooms
- 2 tsps olive oil or sesame oil, plus more for drizzling
- 3 cups (720ml) chicken bone broth or vegetable stock
- 2 tbsps white or brown miso paste
- 1 cooked chicken breast, shredded, or 4 oz (115g) tofu, diced
- 4 leaves of cavolo nero, tough middle stems removed, leaves chopped

PER PORTION + CHICKEN: ✓ 28g protein ✓ 105mg choline
PER PORTION + TOFU: ✓ 12g protein ✓ 65mg choline

- Halve or quarter the **mushrooms**, depending on their size, and tip them into a large saucepan. Add the 2 teaspoons of **olive oil or sesame oil** and cook the mushrooms over medium heat for about 5 minutes, until they are browned and tender.

- Add the **chicken bone broth or vegetable stock** and bring the liquid slowly to a boil. Decrease the heat to a low simmer and cook for about 15 minutes for the mushrooms to infuse the broth.

- Add the **miso** and stir to combine. Then, add the **chicken or tofu** and the **cavolo nero** leaves and cook for 3–4 minutes to heat the chicken or tofu and to wilt the greens. Serve in bowls with a drizzle of olive oil or sesame oil (chile oil is good too).

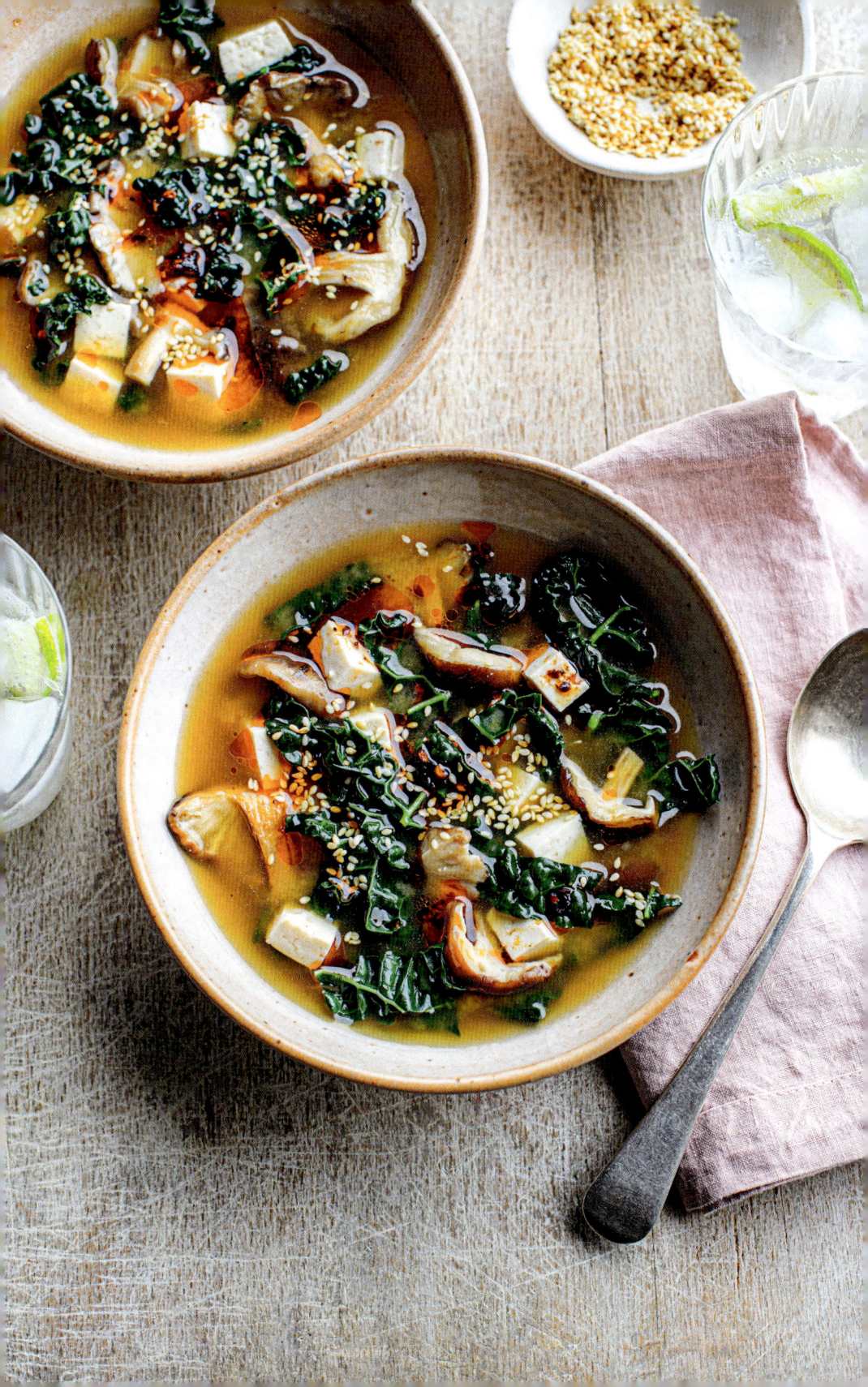

SWEET THINGS

Frozen Yogurt Popsicles

Before you reach for your delivery app and order five tubs of ice cream (been there), why not try this protein-packed and lower-in-sugar alternative? Yes, it takes a little prep and a silicone mold, but the payoff is big. These gorgeous treats live happily in your freezer, ready whenever cravings strike. And if you get that infamous second-trimester energy boost, you could use it to batch a few in advance.

MAKES: 6 POPSICLES

¾ cup (200g) Greek yogurt
Heaped ¾ cup (200g) frozen raspberries or mixed berries (no need to defrost)
1 tbsp honey or maple syrup
1 tsp vanilla extract
1 banana

PER POPSICLE: ✓ 4g protein ✓ 12mg choline

- You will need a 6-hole silicone popsicle mold and 6 popsicle sticks.

- Combine the **yogurt, berries, honey or maple syrup,** and **vanilla** in a high-speed blender. Slice the **banana** into the blender and blend the mixture until smooth.

- Divide the mixture equally among the popsicle molds, filling each one almost to the top. Cover and insert the popsicle sticks. Freeze for 4–6 hours, or until solid. Unmold to serve.

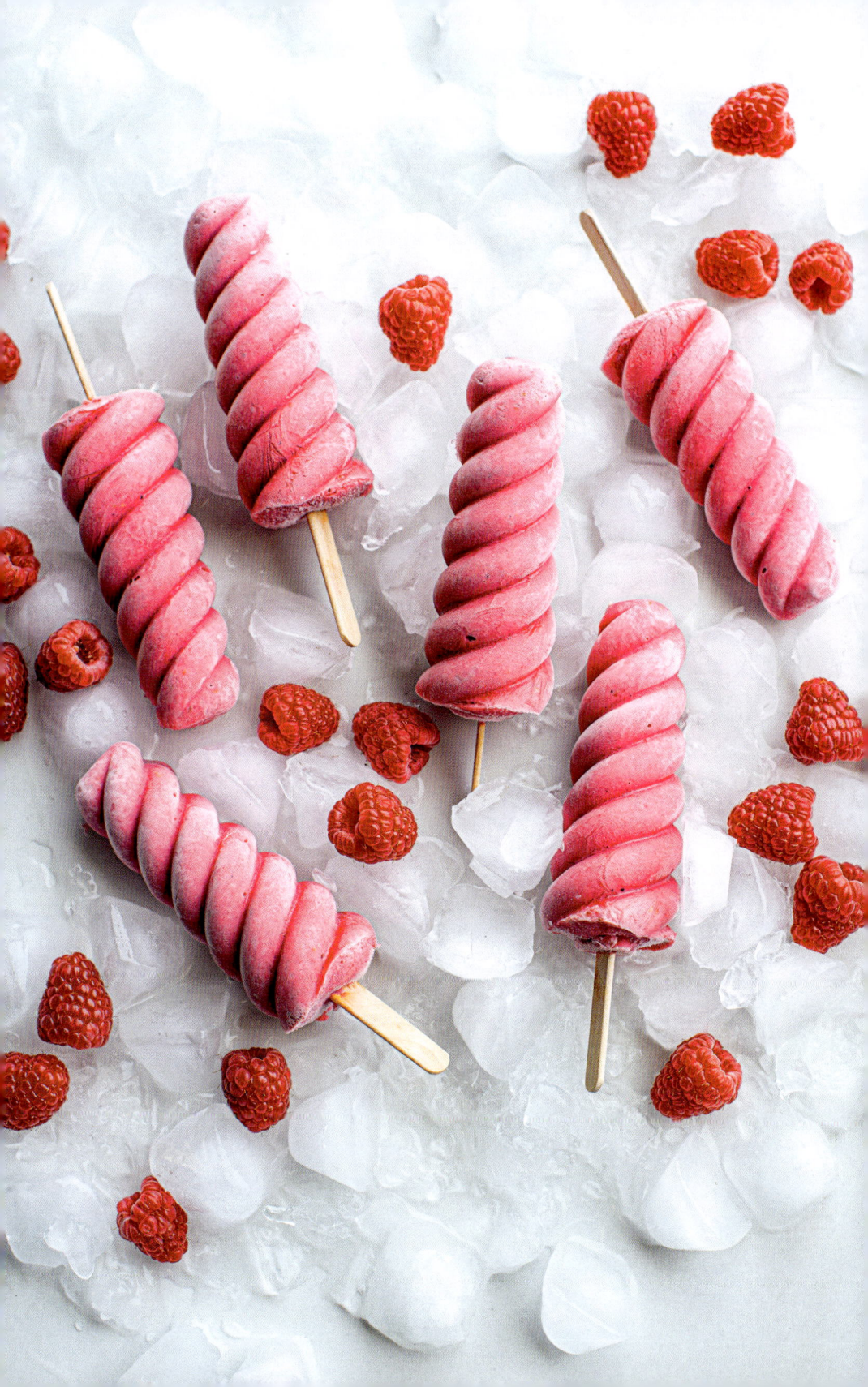

Magic Egg Custard with Plums

Hold up! A sweet dessert, with a ton of choline in it? Is this magic? No, it's just eggs! This is a sweet-treat superpower.

SERVES: 4

6 plums, pitted and halved
juice of ½ a lemon
2 tsps sugar or honey
½ tsp ground cinnamon
3 whole large eggs, plus 1 large yolk

4–6 tbsps (50–75g) sugar
1½ cups (360ml) heavy cream
7 tbsps (100ml) whole milk
½ tsp vanilla bean paste
salt

PER PORTION: ✓ 10g protein ✓ 150mg choline ✓ 30mg DHA (if you use free-range pasture-raised eggs)

- Heat the oven to 350°F. Line a small baking sheet with parchment paper.

- Place the **plums** cut side up on the prepared baking sheet. Sprinkle with the **lemon juice, sugar or honey**, and ground **cinnamon**. Bake the plums for about 30 minutes, until they are juicy and tender. Remove them from the oven and keep them warm, covered with foil, while you prepare the custards.

- Turn the oven temperature down to 300°F and place 4 x ⅔ cup (160ml) capacity ramekins into a small roasting pan.

- In a medium bowl, beat together the **whole eggs, egg yolk**, and **sugar** using a whisk. Add the **heavy cream, whole milk**, and **vanilla bean paste**, along with a pinch of **salt**, and whisk again until smooth and thoroughly combined. Strain the custard mixture through a sieve into a liquid measuring cup and pour it equally into the ramekins to fill them evenly.

- Pour freshly boiled water into the roasting pan around the ramekins so that the water comes halfway up the sides of the pots. Carefully slide the roasting pan into the oven and bake the custards for about 45 minutes until set and piping hot. Remove the roasting pan from the oven and carefully remove the pots from the water.

- Serve the custards immediately, while hot, with the warm plums. The custards will keep covered in the fridge, but be sure to eat them within a day of making, and reheat them to at least 140°F before eating.

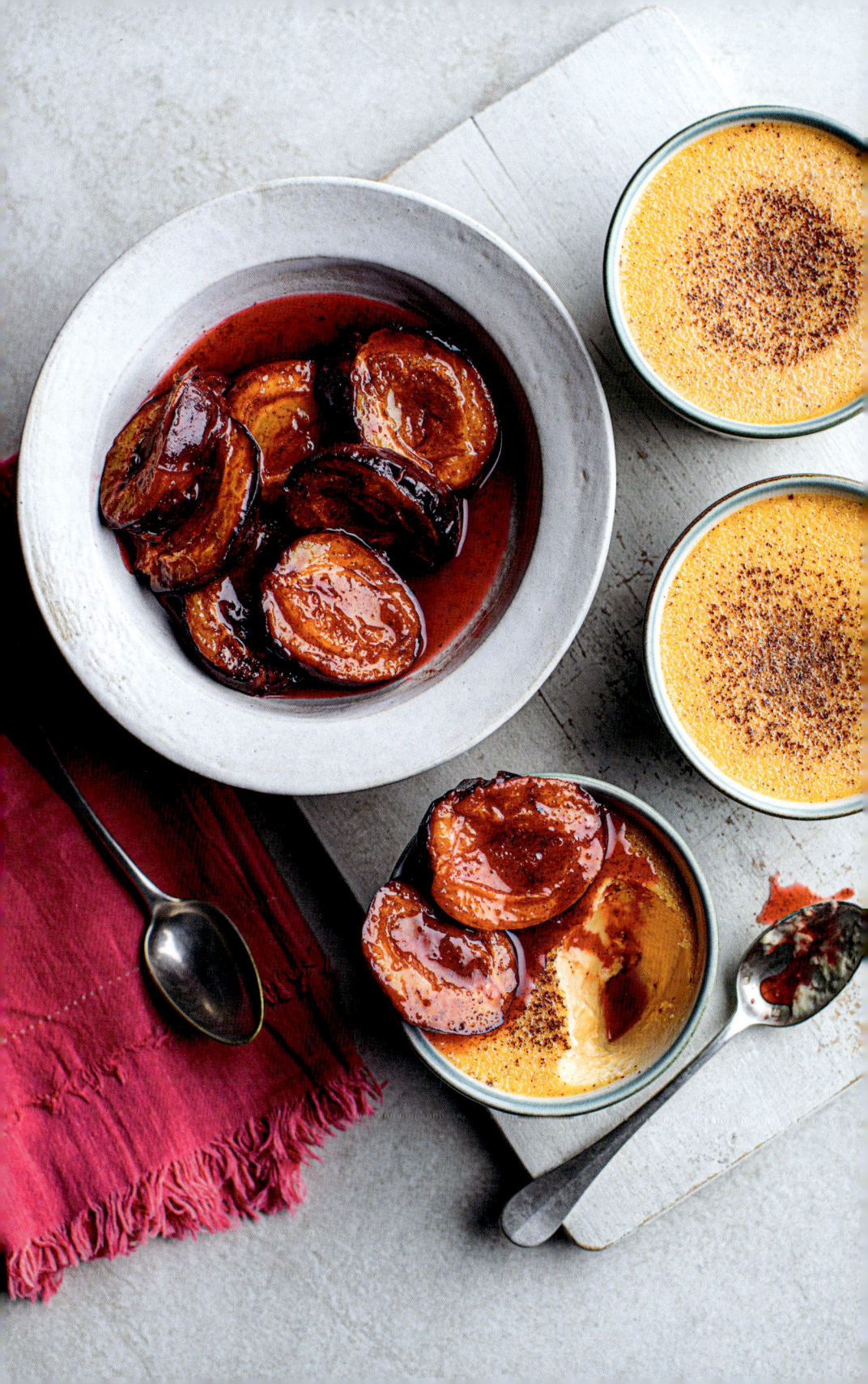

Chocolate Bark

This is a very fun recipe to make. It turns your dark chocolate into something with more pizzazz, and is better for your glucose levels. You can adapt it to include your favorite nuts. Just keep in mind that dark chocolate contains some caffeine, and as pregnancy progresses you will take longer to clear it—a lot of this chocolate bark right before bed might make it harder to fall asleep.

MAKES: 8 PORTIONS

7 oz (200g) 70% dark chocolate
1 tsp extra-virgin olive oil
⅔ cup (90g) nuts (such as hazelnuts, walnuts, pistachios, or almonds), roughly chopped

¼ cup (25g) toasted mixed seeds (pumpkin and sesame work well)
2–3 tsps freeze-dried raspberry pieces or dried cranberries, finely chopped
a good pinch of sea-salt flakes

PER PORTION: ✓ 4g protein ✓ 13mg choline

- Line a rimmed baking sheet with parchment paper.

- Break the **dark chocolate** into pieces and tip it into a heatproof medium bowl. Add the **extra-virgin olive oil** and place the bowl over a saucepan of barely simmering water. Do not allow the bottom of the bowl to touch the water. When the chocolate has almost completely melted, take the bowl off the heat and stir it until smooth. Set aside.

- Spoon the melted chocolate into the prepared baking sheet and, using the back of a spoon, spread it out into a thin layer to an approximately 8 x 12-inch (20 x 30cm) rectangle. Scatter with the chopped **nuts** and toasted **seeds**. Then sprinkle with the **freeze-dried raspberry pieces or dried cranberries** and the **sea-salt flakes**. Sharply tap the bottom of the baking sheet on the work surface to level the chocolate.

- Allow it to set at room temperature for about 2 hours—or, if you can't wait, pop the baking sheet in the fridge for about 30 minutes.

- Once the chocolate has set, break or chop it up into chunks to serve. Store the chocolate pieces in a food container and keep them in the fridge for up to 2 weeks.

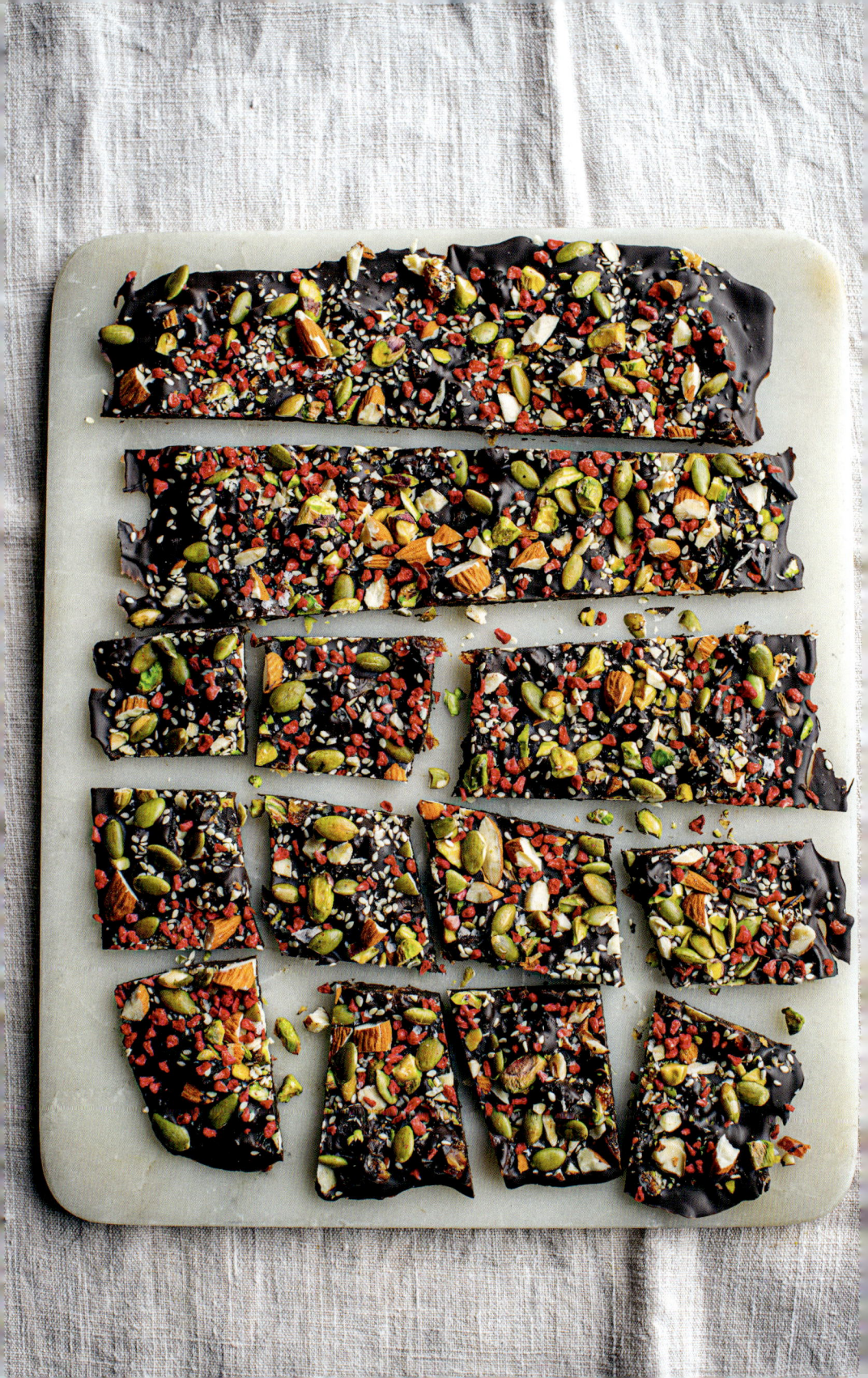

Cheesecake Bites

The trick with this recipe is that it's built around cream cheese and Greek yogurt. The proteins and fats offset the speed at which the sugar will hit your bloodstream. Result? A tasty dessert, and a smaller glucose spike for you and your baby.

SERVES: 6

7 oz (200g) full-fat pasteurized cream cheese
scant ½ cup (125g) Greek yogurt
¼ cup (50g) sugar

1 large egg
1 tsp vanilla bean paste
1 tsp cornstarch

TO SERVE:

⅓ cup (50g) whole, skin-on almonds, finely chopped

fresh berries
seeds and juice from 2–3 passion fruits

PER PORTION: ✓ 6g protein ✓ 40mg choline ✓ 5mg DHA (if you use a free-range pasture-raised egg)

• Heat the oven to 350°F and line a muffin pan with six paper muffin liners.

• In a mixing bowl, combine the **cream cheese, Greek yogurt, sugar, egg,** and **vanilla bean paste** and, using a whisk, mix until smooth. Add the **cornstarch** and mix again until thoroughly combined. Tap the bowl sharply on the work surface to knock out any large air bubbles.

• Spoon the cheesecake mixture equally into the paper liners and spread it level. Bake the cheesecakes for about 20 minutes until set, then let cool. Once cool, chill until you're ready to serve. They will keep up to three days covered in the fridge.

• Serve the cheesecakes with chopped **almonds, fresh berries,** and **passion fruit seeds**.

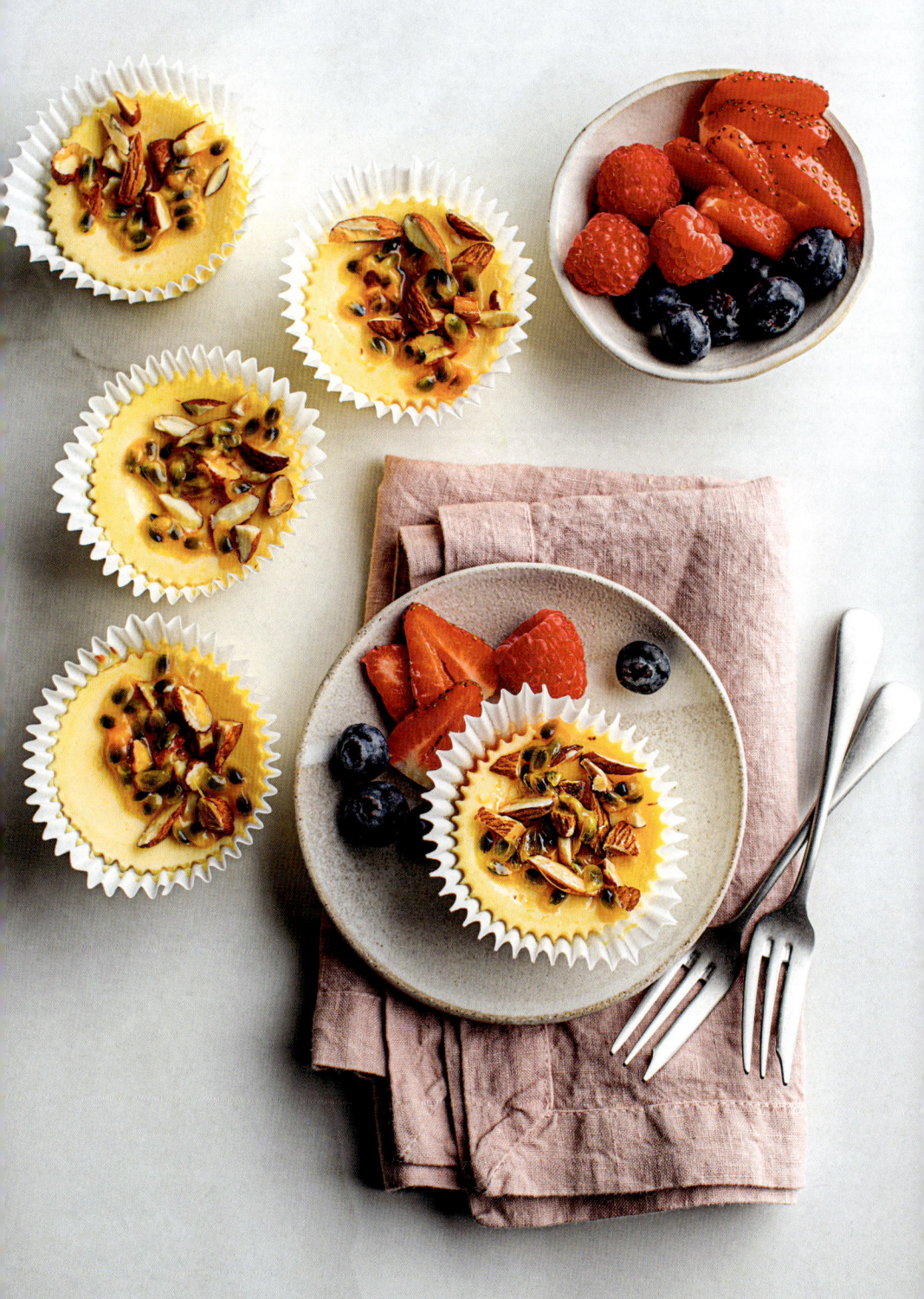

Chocolate Peanut Butter Cups

Last but certainly not least . . . peanut butter and chocolate! You can use peanut or any other nut butter that you prefer in these treats—just make sure to use an unsweetened version (check the ingredients on the back of the jar). These will keep well for a week in the fridge in an airtight food container.

MAKES: 10

10½ oz (300g) 70% or higher dark chocolate
10 tsps (50g) unsweetened peanut butter
⅓ cup (50g) roasted peanuts, roughly chopped
a pinch of sea-salt flakes

PER TRUFFLE: ✓ 7g protein ✓ 14mg choline

- Line a muffin pan with 10 paper muffin liners.

- Break the **chocolate** into chunks and tip it into a heatproof medium bowl. Set the bowl over a saucepan of barely simmering water and allow the chocolate to melt, stirring occasionally until smooth. Don't let the bottom of the bowl touch the water.

- Remove the bowl from the heat, stir the chocolate well until smooth, then let cool for 5 minutes.

- Spoon 1 large spoonful of the melted chocolate into each paper muffin liner and let it cool for 5 minutes. Lift up the pan and gently tilt it from side to side to swirl the chocolate in the paper liner so that it comes up the sides by about 1 inch (2.5cm).

- Spoon 1 teaspoon of **peanut butter** into the middle of each chocolate cup. Cover the peanut butter with the remaining melted chocolate, scatter with **peanuts** and **sea-salt flakes**, and allow the chocolate cups to set in a cool place or in the fridge for 30 minutes.

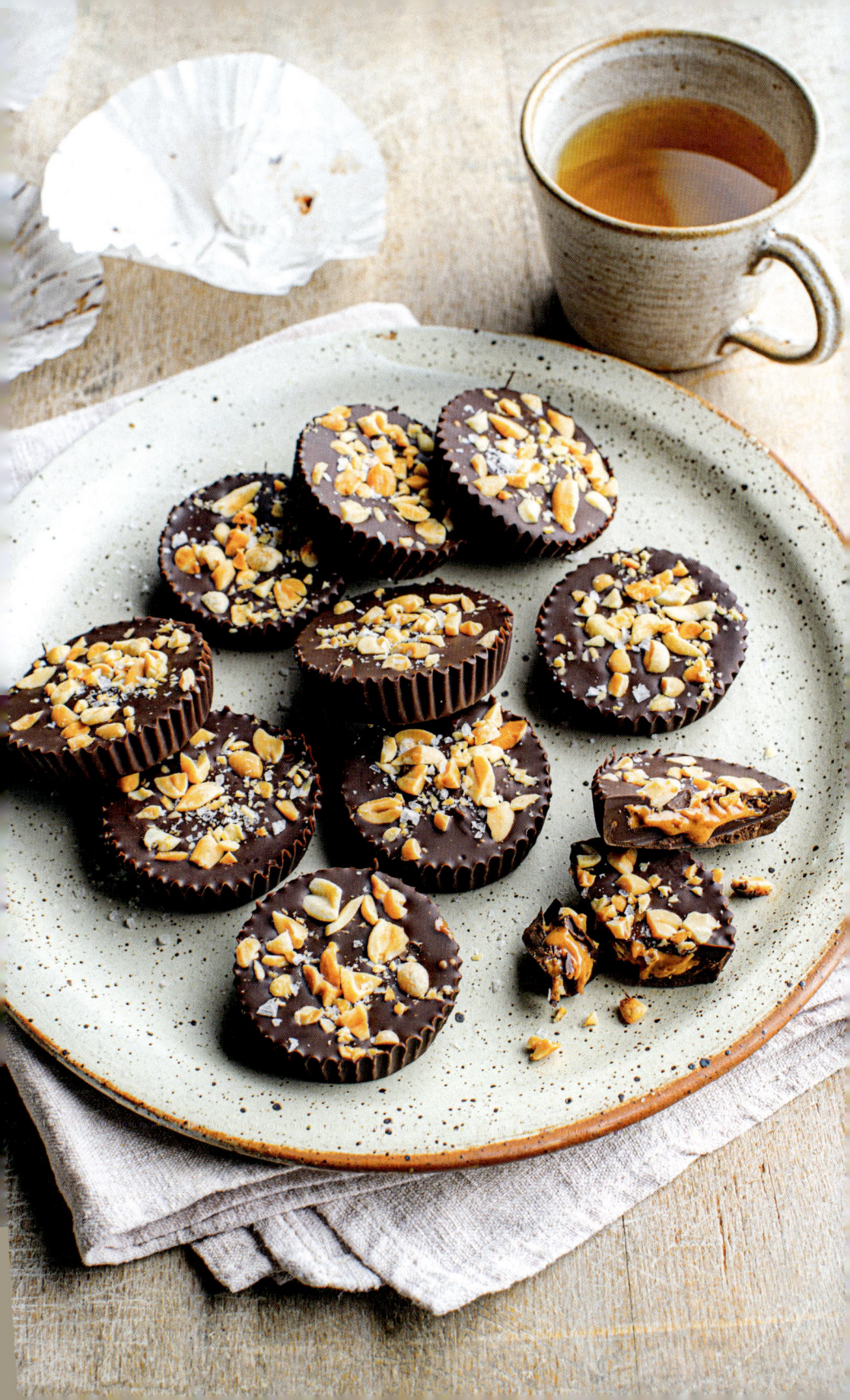

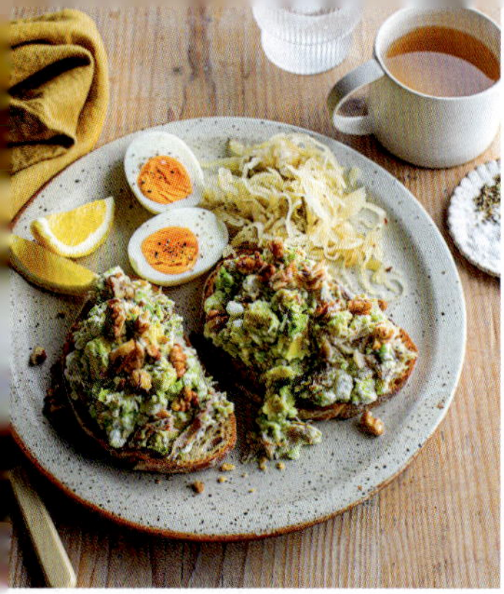

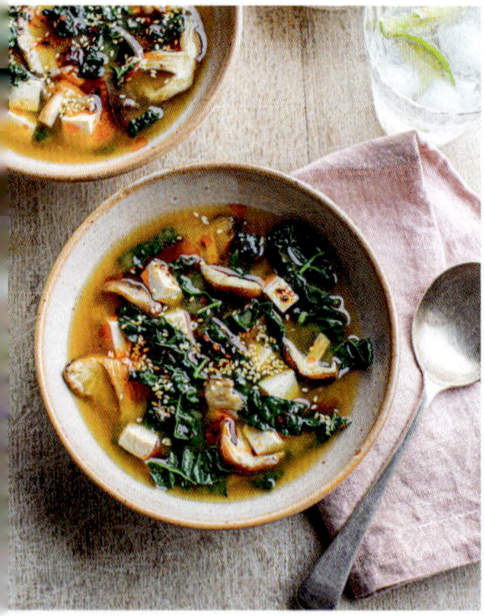

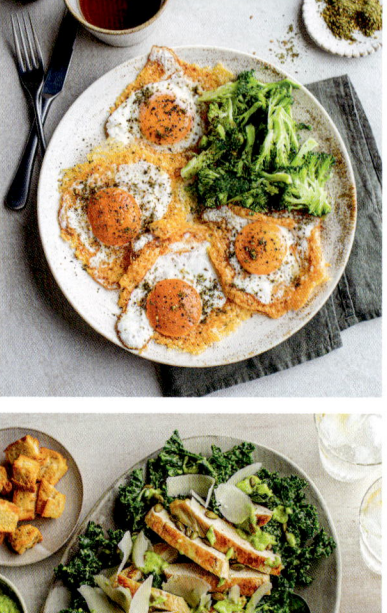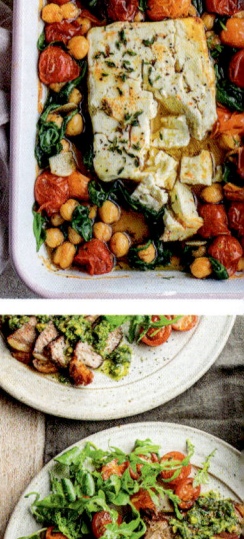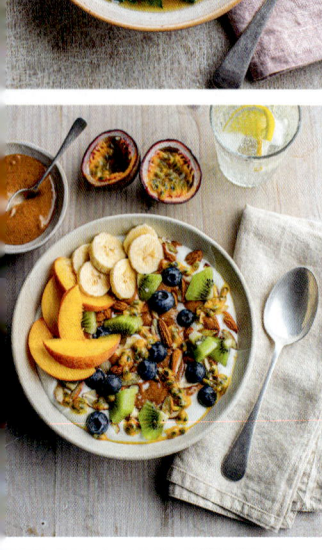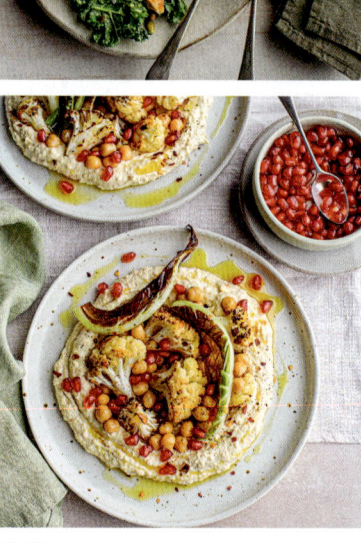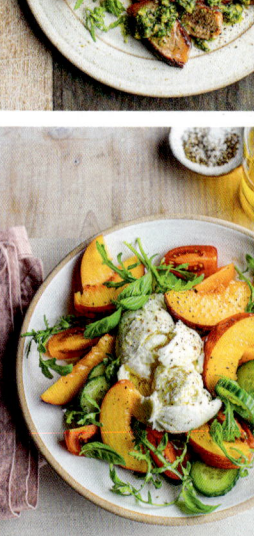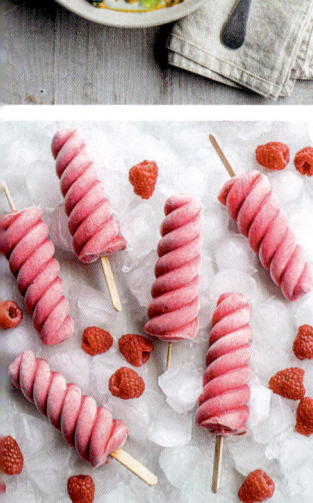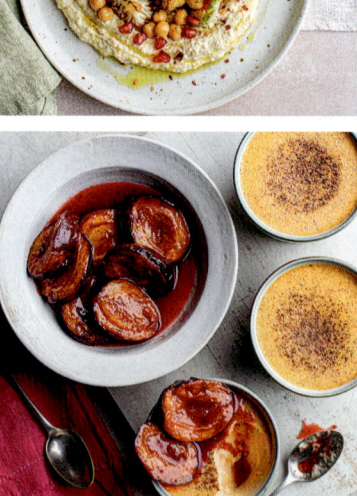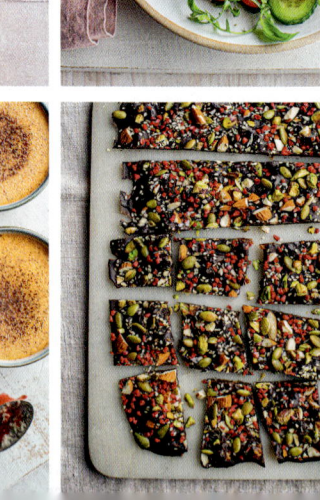